EuropeActive's Essentials for Personal Trainers

EuropeActive

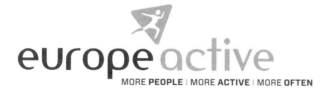

MORE **PEOPLE** I MORE **ACTIVE** I MORE **OFTEN**

Thomas Rieger
Ben Jones
Alfonso Jiménez

EDITORS

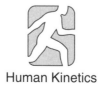

Human Kinetics

Library of Congress Cataloging-in-Publication Data

Names: EuropeActive. | Rieger, Thomas, 1973- editor.
Title: EuropeActive's essentials for personal trainers / EuropeActive ;
   Thomas Rieger, Ben Jones, Alfonso Jimenez, editors.
Description: Champaign, IL : Human Kinetics, [2016] | Includes
   bibliographical references and index.
Identifiers: LCCN 2015041792 | ISBN 9781450423786 (print)
Subjects: LCSH: Personal trainers--Training of--European Union
   countries--Handbooks, manuals, etc. | Personal trainers--Vocational
   guidance--European Union countries--Handbooks, manuals, etc. | Personal
   trainers--Certification--European Union countries--Study guides. |
   Physical education and training--European Union countries--Handbooks,
   manuals, etc.
Classification: LCC GV428.7 .E87 2016 | DDC 613.7/1--dc23 LC record available
   at http://lccn.loc.gov/2015041792

ISBN: 978-1-4504-2378-6 (print)

The web addresses cited in this text were current as of September 2015, unless otherwise noted.

Acquisitions Editor: Roger W. Earle; **Developmental Editor:** Kevin Matz; **Associate Managing Editor:** Shevone Myrick; **Copyeditor:** Joy Hoppenot; **Proofreader:** Jim Burns; **Indexer:** Katy Balcer; **Permissions Manager:** Dalene Reeder; **Senior Graphic Designer:** Nancy Rasmus; **Graphic Designer:** Dawn Sills; **Cover Designer:** Keith Blomberg; **Photographs (interior):** © Human Kinetics, unless otherwise noted; **Photo Asset Manager:** Laura Fitch; **Photo Production Manager:** Jason Allen; **Senior Art Manager:** Kelly Hendren; **Associate Art Manager:** Alan L. Wilborn; **Illustrations:** © Human Kinetics, unless otherwise noted; **Printer:** Edwards Brothers Malloy

Printed in the United States of America   10 9 8 7 6 5 4 3 2 1

The paper in this book is certified under a sustainable forestry program.

Human Kinetics
Website: www.HumanKinetics.com

United States: Human Kinetics
P.O. Box 5076
Champaign, IL 61825-5076
800-747-4457
e-mail: info@hkusa.com

Canada: Human Kinetics
475 Devonshire Road Unit 100
Windsor, ON N8Y 2L5
800-465-7301 (in Canada only)
e-mail: info@hkcanada.com

Europe: Human Kinetics
107 Bradford Road
Stanningley
Leeds LS28 6AT, United Kingdom
+44 (0) 113 255 5665
e-mail: hk@hkeurope.com

Australia: Human Kinetics
57A Price Avenue
Lower Mitcham, South Australia 5062
08 8372 0999
e-mail: info@hkaustralia.com

New Zealand: Human Kinetics
P.O. Box 80
Mitcham Shopping Centre, South Australia 5062
0800 222 062
e-mail: info@hknewzealand.com

E5641

Contents

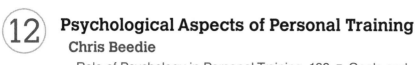

Psychological Aspects of Personal Training   189

Chris Beedie

Nutrition   203

Fernando Naclerio and Robert Cooper

PART V   Training Adaptations, Exercise Planning and Programming

Training Adaptations   227

Rafael Oliveira, João Brito and Ben Jones

Exercise Planning and Programming   241

Christoffer Andersen, Thomas Rieger
and Lars L. Andersen

Preface

Personal training is undoubtedly one of the most important occupations in the European fitness industry. The job market for personal trainers currently shows excellent opportunities because obese and ailing populations now understand the need for fitness, nutrition and an active lifestyle. Accordingly both the number of exercise professionals with personal trainer certification and training providers offering such courses are steadily increasing. A significant majority of accredited training providers in Europe have decided to make their personal training courses applicable for the EuropeActive accreditation. Most of the professionals on the European Register of Exercise Professionals (EREPS) hold a personal trainer qualification. Nevertheless compared to the U.S. market, there is still room for growth and development in Europe. The U.S. government's Bureau of Labor Statistics predicts a 29 percent increase in exercise professionals between 2008 and 2018. In other words the personal trainer occupation is a success story. Based on a shift in societal values, there is more demand for individualised services like personal training. Consumers want to be addressed personally in order to ensure optimal conditions for achieving their physical and health-related goals. Personal trainers have the skills, competency and knowledge to fulfil these expectations. As mentioned before the relevance of this profession is reflected in the European educational standards for fitness developed by the Standards Council of EuropeActive and its experts. At the moment the European Qualifications Framework (EQF) includes the following formally published standards for all vocational levels: fitness assistant (EQF level 2), fitness and group fitness instructor (EQF level 3), personal trainer, active ageing trainer, youth fitness instructor, Pilates teacher (all EQF level 4), and exercise for health specialist, (pre)diabetes exercise specialist and weight management exercise specialist (all EQF level 5).

The EQF links the qualifications systems of countries in Europe, acting as a translation device to make qualifications more understandable. This will help learners and workers wishing to

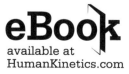

eBook
available at
HumanKinetics.com

move between countries, change jobs or move between educational institutions at home.

The series reflects the current status of educational fitness standards in Europe and provides the foundations at EQF level 2, following with the essentials for fitness instructors at EQF level 3 and for personal trainers at EQF level 4.

With regard to the number of accredited training programmes based on these standards, it becomes obvious that personal trainer courses play a key role in this context. Hence after the publication of *EuropeActive's Foundations for Exercise Professionals* (EQF level 2) and *EuropeActive's Essentials for Fitness Instructors* (EQF level 3), EuropeActive and Human Kinetics have decided to continue this series with this textbook, *EuropeActive's Essentials for Personal Trainers* (EQF level 4).

EuropeActive's Essentials for Personal Trainers provides a standard reference for teaching the basic competencies, skills and knowledge that personal trainers need. The book is divided into the following parts and chapters: The Role of the Personal Trainer (chapters 1 through 3: Professionalism and Presentation, Planning a Personal Training Session, Delivering a Personal Training Session), Functional Anatomy (chapters 4 through 6: Skeletal Articulations and Joint Movement, Injury Prevention, Muscular System), Physiology (chapters 7 through 10: Energy Systems, Cardiorespiratory System, Nervous System, Hormonal Responses to Exercise), Lifestyle Assessment (chapters 11 through 13: Health and Fitness Assessment, Psychological Aspects of Personal Training, Nutrition) and Training Adaptations, Exercise Planning and Programming (chapters 14 and 15: Training Adaptations, Exercise Planning and Programming).

Personal trainers should be acquainted with the skills, competencies and knowledge from the aforementioned fields, since they are based on a very comprehensive process of standards development set by EuropeActive's Standards Council and supported by the commitment of many renowned exercise and fitness experts worldwide. The textbook is primarily aimed at exercise professionals serving as personal trainers. In addition training providers can use it as the basic teaching material within their personal trainer courses to assure that their course is in line with the current standards. This textbook gives a perfect orientation for what is needed to successfully apply for EuropeActive accreditation. Finally *EuropeActive's Essentials for Personal Trainers* is also intended for personal trainers, coaches, students of sports and exercise science as well as anyone who is interested in exercising, fitness, physical activity and health. The content bundled in this book ideally prepares personal trainers all over the world to deliver client-oriented service grounded on current research. As always we are trying to get more people more active, more often. Hence, this is the must-have textbook for personal trainers across Europe and beyond.

The Standards Council of EuropeActive sincerely thanks all those who have been involved in this project, especially the editors and authors for their willingness to contribute.

Prof. Dr. Thomas Rieger
Chairman of EuropeActive's Standards Council
Brussels, September 2015

The Role of the
Personal Trainer →→→

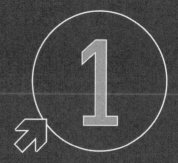

Professionalism and Presentation

Jan Middelkamp

The purpose of this chapter is to set a framework for the profession of personal training in Europe. Although this segment of the European fitness industry is growing quickly, little is known about personal training. Basic data are lacking on the amount of personal trainers, their clients and quality of the profession in general. This chapter discusses several issues connected with personal training, including definitions of personal training, profiles of personal trainers and personal training clients, and many general items related to the business of personal training.

Personal Training

Personal training is a generic name for a palette of activities. Call it a container term, because almost everything fits inside. The broad character of personal training has advantages and disadvantages, beauty and flaws. The pluralism of this term and the related discipline offers room for various angles and shapes, with many practices and meanings to choose from. However, this versatility also creates obscurities and confusion, and can lead to disappointments for the clients. The American College of Sports Medicine (ACSM 2007) defines personal training this way: 'The ACSM Certified personal trainer is a fitness professional involved in developing and implementing an individualised approach to exercise leadership in healthy populations and/or those individuals with medical clearance to exercise. Using a variety of teaching techniques, the ACSM Certified personal trainer is proficient in leading and demonstrating safe and effective methods of exercise by applying the fundamental principles of exercise science. The ACSM Certified personal trainer is proficient in writing appropriate exercise recommendations, leading and demonstrating safe and effective methods of exercise, and motivating individuals to begin and to continue with their healthy behaviours' (p. 5). Earle and Baechle (2003) further describe what personal trainers do: 'A personal trainer is a fitness professional involved in exercise prescription and instruction. They motivate clients by setting goals and providing feedback and accountability to clients. Personal trainers also measure their client's strengths and weaknesses with fitness assessments. These fitness assessments may also be performed before and after an exercise program to measure their client's improvements in physical fitness. They may also educate their clients in many other aspects of wellness besides exercise, including general health and nutrition guidelines. Qualified personal trainers recognise their own areas of expertise. If a personal trainer suspects that one of his or her clients has a medical condition that could prevent the client from safe participation in an exercise program, they must refer the client to the proper health professional for prior clearance' (p. 6).

Definitions like these mainly describe what the profession of a personal trainer should encompass according to the organisation or author concerned. As always, all definitions are open for discussion, and each has pros and cons. Note, for example, the fact that a personal trainer does not explicitly have to perform a paid activity (provide fee-based services). In Europe, personal training is still a relatively new phenomenon for the fitness industry in general and for consumers in particular. However it is a growing profession. What should a consumer expect of a personal trainer? And when is a person qualified to use the label of personal trainer? The answers to questions like these are important for accurately matching demand with supply. This process is still in its infancy in Europe and in other continents, which is partly due to the broad interpretation given to the profession of personal training.

Profiles of Personal Trainers and Clients

Little factual information (i.e., research) is available about personal training. Yet, experiences and impressions are intensively discussed in the sector. For instance, a commonly heard statistic is that roughly 50 percent of personal trainers throw in the towel within 12 months of starting the profession. It is unknown where this knowledge comes from, or whether it differs among kinds of personal trainer and different countries. Generally speaking we know very little about this discipline and its players. The following section briefly discusses profiles of personal trainers and their clients.

A profile of personal trainers emerged from research conducted by Horn (2011) on personal training in Germany. The personal trainers from Horn's study have an average age of 36 years old, with a variation of 22 to 59 years. The majority of personal trainers in Germany are men (60 percent) and are highly educated, often in *Sportwissenschaft* (exercise science). Horn's study showed that the proportion of personal trainers who practise their trade full-time versus part-time is changing. In 2004, 55 percent of trainers worked full-time and 45 percent part-time; in 2011, 66 percent worked full-time and only 34 percent part-time. Thirteen percent worked as part of a team in a fitness club. In Germany, full-time personal trainers earn 3,200 euros net a month on average. Melton, Katula and Mustian (2008) studied the personal trainers' perception of factors that determine success. In their study, four main groups are prominent: the considerations of clients when choosing a personal trainer, the loyalty of clients, education, and negative characteristics. In the first group, the physical appearance of the personal trainer seems to be most important, followed by sex, race and niche (here it is important that the personal trainer can meet the specific needs of a certain client) and referral (recommendations from other clients). With regard to the loyalty of clients, personal trainers believe that motivational skills, individuality (this concerns the ability of the personal trainer to make the client feel special), empathic abilities and social skills are important. A follow-up study from Melton and colleagues (2010) describes the views of managers about the necessary qualities of a personal trainer. The most notable result is that managers label the physical appearance of the personal trainers as especially important.

Little is known from research about clients or potential clients of personal trainers. Of course personal trainers know all details and profiles of their own clients, but a more general picture is lacking. Kronsteiner (2010) conducted a small study that provides some information on clients of personal trainers. The average age of the client sample is 43 years old. It is notable that club members who train with a personal trainer were older than members training without a personal trainer: 48 years old versus 37 years old. In Horn's study (2011), 58 percent of the personal training clients were between 36 and 45 years old. Merely 4 percent of clients were younger than 35. In both studies (Horn and Kronsteiner), the largest group of clients of personal trainers consisted of entrepreneurs and self-employed earners. In Kronsteiner's study (2010), no less than 42 percent of the clientele was self-employed. Additionally, many clients are managers. A striking third group are pensioners (11 percent). Among personal training clients, 51 percent had a university education, compared to 43 percent of the non-personal training clients in the same club. Unfortunately little can be said about personal training in Europe in general on the basis of empirical research. EuropeActive wants to take important steps to further define the discipline of personal training and aims to collect and publish more information on personal training in order to intensively develop this discipline. The objective of this chapter is to sketch a further picture of the discipline of personal training in Europe. This chapter gives special attention to themes such as professionalism in general and presentation in particular.

Examining the Sector of Personal Training

The average consumer may struggle to understand what personal training is. People often associate training with physical exercise, but training can also take place on a mental level. Personal training comprises more than just physical exercise; for example, it includes nutritional coaching. Exercise or training may be the principal part, but it is certainly not the only part. Due to the philosophy that the customer is king, personal training is interpreted in a multitude of ways. The place or setting where personal training takes place is also diverse. Table 1.1 provides a concise overview of settings of personal training, giving a brief overview of the characteristics of different settings both from the client's perspective and the personal trainer's perspective (Middelkamp and Willemsen 2010).

Every setting of personal training has its own particular characteristics. If we summarise the items from the preceding table, matters such as flexibility, facilities, travel time, investment (for the personal trainer) and experience value are especially important. Both the client and the personal trainer should make their choices based on these factors. These factors can help personal trainers realise a market position. When, for instance, all personal trainers work from a fitness club in a town, a few could position themselves well by offering home sessions. All in all this range of choices offers a multitude of opportunities for everyone involved. The client has options, but the personal trainers and even the fitness club owners do as well. Clubs are also able to offer a diversity of options, naturally using the club as starting point.

Following its success in the United States, small group personal training (SGPT) is increasingly in demand in Europe. A large number of well-known forms of training and methods are offered in small-

Table 1.1 Settings of Personal Training

Setting	Client's perspective	Personal trainer's perspective
At the client's home	Comfortable environment No travel time Fewer facilities Generally more expensive	Some or even considerable travel time and expenses Optimal service Bringing personal materials or using client's materials
In the fitness club	Little privacy A lot of facilities Social environment	A lot of facilities Large clientele base Possibly more immediate competition of fellow personal trainers
At work or in hotel	Matches well with planning and schedule Generally more expensive	Some or even considerable time and expenses Optimal service
Outdoor (e.g., beach, forest)	Special/high experience value Extra clothes possibly necessary	Risk: less control of environment Sometimes requires transport of materials
At the personal trainer's camper	No travel time High flexibility	Requires some investment Provides flexibility Distinguishing strategy
In personal training studio	Requires travel time, just as with clubs More facilities More privacy than in a club	Requires significant investment A lot of facilities
Online via the Internet	Easy access A lot of privacy A lot of distance, little personal contact	Can reach a lot of clients without too much effort Little personal contact

Reprinted, by permission, from J. Middelkamp and G. Willemsen, eds., 2010, *Personal training in Europa* (Waalwijk, Netherlands: LAPT).

group format, or in groups of two to eight people. A fee-based construction is, for instance, charging each client 9 euros for a 30-minute session with a group of six people. The turnover for the personal trainer is 54 euros per half hour in this case. For the personal trainer, the SGPT variation offers an interesting variation to the one-to-one sessions. It often generates higher income per hour. For the clients, SGPT offers a more affordable option and a higher social factor.

Business Models of Personal Training

Both a fitness club and a personal trainer should think about how they would like to offer personal training. This choice is largely determined by a commercial perspective, but personal or organisational elements also play a role. Roughly three business models exist, and

Table 1.2 Overview of Personal Training Business Models

Model	Characteristics
Employee	Personal trainer on club's payroll Turnover goes to club Personal trainer often receives a commission per session
Licence	Personal trainer is an independent entrepreneur Turnover goes to personal trainer Club supports personal trainer with a multitude of facilities Club receives licence fee (part rent and part payment for licence facilities)
Rent	Personal trainer is independent Turnover goes to personal trainer Personal trainers pay rent and define their own way of working Personal trainers take care of everything themselves (including their own personal training materials)

a few subforms can be distinguished (table 1.2). Each model has its own characteristics (Middelkamp and Willemsen 2010).

The licence model is sometimes also called the franchise model. The exact difference is difficult to point out, but franchising seems to be more complicated legally and more comprehensive. In some cases, the licenser or franchiser provides the personal trainer with a multitude of opportunities, such as their own brand, marketing support, training, workshops and joint purchase. Within the licence model personal trainers have two additional options: doing the work themselves or outsourcing to an external licenser. The first option is unrealistic for a single fitness club, but possibly doable for a fitness chain with a large number of clubs. For a fitness club, the choice for a model has far-reaching consequences (see the following list for an overview).

Consequences of Personal Training Business Models From the Fitness Club's Perspective

- Employee model
  - High personnel expenses
  - More management activities
  - Turnover goes to the club
  - Relatively high turnover
  - High control over quality
  - A lot of cross-contamination (e.g., on retention)
- Licence model
  - No personnel expenses
  - Little management activities

- □ Relatively low turnover
- □ Turnover goes to the personal trainer
- □ Reasonable control over quality
- □ Less cross-contamination
- ■ Rent model
  - □ No personnel expenses
  - □ Little management activities
  - □ Low turnover (rent)
  - □ Turnover goes to the personal trainer
  - □ Virtually no control over quality
  - □ Less cross-contamination

For a personal trainer, choosing a certain model has consequences. The rent model actually requires more entrepreneurship because personal trainers have to arrange everything themselves. Think about general conditions, website, purchase, payment traffic and administration. In the licence model personal trainers receive significantly more support, for instance, central education, purchasing and exchange of materials such as general conditions and operational forms. A beginning personal trainer often starts from a paid employment model. This occurs on a large scale with fitness instructors. Starting from a paid employment model offers personal trainers more safety and security. The income, on the other hand, is lower than with independent entrepreneurship. Employed personal trainers who have built up the necessary experience sometimes take the step to become independent entrepreneurs, which usually brings them more freedom and more income.

Quality Perspectives in Personal Training

With respect to the theme of professionalism a logical question is, what is quality? Or differently phrased, what characterises a good personal trainer? Countless factors determine the success of a personal trainer. The perspective from which the question is posed is crucial. Is this from the point of view of the client, the club or the personal trainer? Or of all of them? At first sight a good or great personal trainer is simply one who realises the goals of their clients in a safe way and for the long term. But other important matters must be considered in addition to these main objectives. Table 1.3 briefly summarises these by means of four quality perspectives: the quality of the product and the process, as well as the value for the client and society.

In a healthy personal training situation, product quality and client satisfaction should be accurately tuned in to each other. Therefore they appear to be similar. However they differ in certain situations,

Table 1.3   Quality Perspectives With Personal Training

Quality	Dimension	Process	Aspects with personal training
Internal quality	Product quality	Delivery according to the specifications	Expertise First aid knowledge and skills Network of specialists Quality training materials
	Process quality	Delivery is made according to the specifications in an efficient and effective way	Immaculate administrations Good distribution of working week Limited travel time and expenses Overview of turnover and expenses
External quality	Value for the client	The product matches the client's expectations	Client achieves result Save training Service Flexibility Confidential treatment of info
	Value for society	The product and the product process meet societal expectations	No doping Health effects No damaging environmental effects

Reprinted, by permission, from J. Lucassen, M. Van Bottenburg, and J. Van Hoecke, 2006, *Kwaliteitsmanagement in de sport,* 2nd ed. (Nieuwegein, Netherlands: Arko, SportsMedia).

for instance, with a personal trainer who possesses all the required (scientific) knowledge and skills in the field of exercise, but is weak in social skills, communication and motivational strategies. If this personal trainer has a client who deems the social and communicative side to be of great importance, that person can value their experience with the personal trainer as poor. Imagine that a personal trainer provides top-quality training, and the client also experiences it as such. The client achieves training results. However the personal trainer sends inaccurate bills that are too high time and time again. The process quality is clearly not okay. As a result the personal trainer can lose their status as well as countless clients. The process quality is also poor when the personal trainer has clients in Brussels, Amsterdam and Paris and therefore has extremely long travel times. The personal trainer will notice this in their income.

Societal issues are not considered nearly enough in the field. The use of doping substances is a typical example for personal trainers. The client could achieve a quick result using these, but nevertheless personal trainers must not work with these drugs. The use of doping is illegal, unhealthy and unacceptable in the personal training practice.

Professionalism of Personal Trainers in Business

The profession of personal trainer differs from other positions in the fitness industry, including that of fitness instructor, in many ways. More professional activity and entrepreneurship is demanded of personal trainers, whether they are employed by a club or own a business. Personal trainers in paid employment often handle clients differently. More flexibility is demanded, and their salary is often variable. The way a fitness professional communicates with clients is substantially different in the job of fitness instructor. The differences between personal trainers and fitness instructors follow:

1. Personal trainers are focused only on their clients. This means 100 percent focus. This can be one-to-one work, but can also include a small group of four to six people. During the session personal trainers do not have interruptions. In contrast fitness instructors generally have to divide their time across a large number of clients or members.

2. Personal trainers are completely dedicated to realising the goals of their clients. An average personal trainer has roughly 20 to 30 clients. This means complete dedication, but also high dependence. A personal trainer puts the client objectives first and does everything to realise these. Personal training is definitely not just about 60-minute training sessions. It also includes matters such as coaching in terms of nutrition (for instance, creating a grocery list), mental coaching and coaching online or by telephone.

3. A personal trainer should be very flexible. The personal trainer arranges to meet when it is convenient for the client. In regular fitness coaching, everything is tuned to the possibilities in the work schedule. The personal trainer is more flexible, and can even do a training session outside the club, late at night or early in the morning.

4. A personal trainer is supposed to know more and be able to do more than the average fitness instructor. Most personal trainers have been fitness instructors for years, but they have frequently updated their skills and knowledge. Many possess special qualities that help clients achieve their health and fitness goals better and faster. Within the field of personal training, specialising is essential. A professional

personal trainer never pretends to be good at everything. What you win in depth, you automatically lose in width, and vice versa.

5. A personal trainer performs other exercises with their clients. A personal trainer has more space, possibilities and materials for making training more functional, because they mostly work one-to-one. Functional training simply means that personal trainers provide exercises that better fit the daily life situations of the client.

Due to these differences, personal trainers should reflect on their views, mission, goals and passion. This becomes even more important when the number of personal trainers in the market increases. Why would a client opt for one specific personal trainer over another?

Growth Scenarios

To guarantee the result for clients, beginning personal trainers should carefully program growth per week. Personal trainers in paid employment do not usually determine this schedule themselves, although independent personal trainers naturally do. In any case, personal trainers should deliberately choose their growth scenario, and should always plan for the long term. A steady growth scenario creates space for 100 percent focus and 100 percent results with the current clients. This is the foundation of personal training.

In a 40-week growth scenario, the novice personal trainer receives only one new client a week (who schedules two or three sessions per week). The first week begins with one client who is maximally coached. If necessary, the personal trainer gives extra sessions or extra advice over the phone or by text message, to positively influence the client's training results. If the personal trainer and the personal training manager perceive that the client is reporting real results, the personal trainer gets an extra client. So in week 2, the personal trainer coaches two clients, and so on.

A more experienced (but still fairly new) personal trainer can be placed in the 20-week scenario, receiving two new clients every week: week 1, two clients; week 2, four clients; week 3, six clients, and so on. At 10 weeks, this personal trainer will be fully booked because with 20 clients, they will deliver 30 to 35 sessions per week. Of course this is an idealistic scenario in which the personal trainer takes the best possible care of clients, but the central idea is clear: quality first, quantity second.

It is of course not simple to determine when a novice personal trainer should take the next step (extra clients in the next week). The scenarios do not have to be applied literally; they can be adjusted along the way. The real training result may also not be determined on a weekly basis. Both the client and the personal trainer are better off with steady growth. Some fitness chains use this philosophy and thus restrict the number of clients that their personal trainers work with, keeping their numbers between 15 and 20 clients or 25 to 35 sessions per week. For them, taking on a greater number of clients is simply not possible because it would negatively influence the quality of the programme.

Maturity Scenarios

In the end, every personal trainer chooses their own career on the basis of personal situation, objectives and preferences. It is wonderful that personal training offers all sorts of options for this. Experience shows that personal trainers in Europe often started as fitness instructors in paid employment. Successful personal trainers often opt to next make the step to independent entrepreneurship. The career of the personal trainer in the direction of more independence can include several steps (see table 1.4).

A personal trainer has a possible growth scenario from part-time to full-time, and from being an employee with a fixed-base salary to having more variable pay. With variable pay the personal trainer runs a risk. The reward in the form of a commission has to be significantly higher than the risk with less variability. Subsequently the personal trainer can choose to take the step towards being an independent entrepreneur using either the rent model or the licence model.

A successful personal trainer will quickly fill up their hours each week. A personal trainer delivers approximately 25 to 35 sessions per week. The remaining time is required for matters such as service,

Table 1.4   Career Steps for Personal Trainers

Model	Possible steps in career
Personal trainer in paid employment	With 100% base salary
	With smaller base salary and part commission
	With low or no base salary and high commission
	Personal trainer manager
Personal trainer with a licence in the same club	All turnover goes to the personal trainer
	Personal trainer pays club licence fee
	Turnover grows by higher hourly fee (among other causes)
Personal trainer expands business and hires other personal trainers	Possibly attract personal trainers as independent contractors
	Possibly attract personal trainers and hire them as paid employees

sales, administration and travelling. When a personal trainer is fully booked, the first strategy is to increase the price per session. This is especially true for new clients. Existing clients have agreements that can be adjusted only after a certain time. Using session cards with a shorter group of sessions, such as a package of 6 to 12 sessions, can be advantageous. Because the package ends sooner than a club membership, there are more opportunities to adjust the price. For loyal clients this does not happen often in practice. A simple hint is to always adjust the prices at the beginning of the year (January 1st). This can be done with the use of the consumer price index. This minimal increase is applied to account for inflation, because other-wise the personal trainer earns less money. Such matters should be mentioned in the general conditions in any case. A personal trainer can also earn more with small group personal training sessions. With a group of four people, where every client pays 39 euros an hour, a personal trainer earns 136 euros per hour (after deducting GVA).

Experienced personal trainers will not have a problem selling 6- or 12-session packages. The continuity these packages offer is obviously lower than with packages of two sessions per week for at least 6 months (52 sessions). It is a greater challenge to sell a client a personal training subscription of a year's coaching with two sessions per week. At an hourly rate of 75 euros (including GVA), 45 active weeks per year and two sessions per week, the client buys a package worth 6,750 euros. Some clients will pay this in cash. Others prefer to pay by direct debit each month (562.50 euros). Some personal trainers sell long-term packages like these each day, which not only earn them more money, but also provide a better continuity for their business. Continuity is exactly what is often missing for personal trainers. This situation is not unique to personal trainers. Many self-employed people are in the same situation. However it is far from desirable. Ideally personal trainers should build up a business that they could eventually sell, even though they might never wish to sell it.

From One-Person Business to a Steady Company

An important prosperity scenario is expanding a personal training business by employing multiple personal trainers. This is possible by hiring them as employees or by connecting them to the business as self-employed contractors. Naturally the consequences differ greatly. The risk is significantly higher if an entrepreneur hires one or more personal trainers. However the income is also higher. The relationship between base salary and commission can be managed. Little specific information is present on the criteria for hiring someone or expanding the team. A good principle is to not grow and mature too soon. It is better to first build on the strategies mentioned previously before switching to having a lot of employees. So, an entrepreneur should first increase turnover per hour and then try to build up continuity with subscriptions for personal training. When working with a team, usually a small team of two to six people, the entrepreneur should make sure to divide the core tasks efficiently, making sure that not everyone does the same thing, namely delivering sessions. Specialise the team in terms of two issues. The first concerns content: Make sure that every member has their own specialty, or better yet assemble a team of personal trainers with complementary specialties. The second concerns the commercial dimension. Hire a few trainers who continuously recruit new clients in addition to delivering sessions. In this way the entrepreneur will work intensively on the growth of new clients.

An entrepreneur should preferably work on the business instead of just in the business. Ideally a personal trainer who starts their own business should be working on this process from the very beginning. They should strive to make the business saleable, whether or not that is the ultimate intention. This approach has not been applied often in personal training. Why should personal trainers strive to make their business saleable when they have not yet envisioned this goal? They are just getting started. The crux is in the long-term view. Personal trainers are just getting started when they're only 25 or 35 years old, but what about when they are 55 or 65 years old? Since the profession is also very physical, personal trainers need to think ahead about age from the beginning of their careers. But long-term planning is not just about the physical aspects of the profession. The business perspectives might even be more important. A successful personal trainer has added value and made profit in the first years. That is step one. Step two concerns ensuring continuity. When a personal trainer grows value in the first year (e.g., more sessions, more turnover per session), it is a shame when that value stays at the same level for decades afterwards. In all business, an important goal is to continuously raise the economic value of the company. Of course an individual personal trainer could decide explicitly to not strive for this, but it is advised from a long-term business perspective. When personal trainers embrace this growth strategy, they must set up management systematically. They will need a *customer relationship management* (CRM) system to ensure mutual tuning, to build up a database and to obtain reports. They should also ensure matching between methods so that clients do not experience large differences between personal trainers.

These processes are crucial when personal trainers strive to make their business saleable. No one will buy a business when its turnover completely depends on one or two people. A business as an entity has value only when there is continuity. This is true for turnover, profit and all other matters; some are mentioned in the following list:

1. Build a brand. This should not be linked to one person. It has to be an entity that is presented everywhere.
2. Work with a CRM system to record processes and register matters such as client information and make financial data clear.
3. Keep tight control of all financial processes. Never work in undeclared employment. This creates a wrong image towards the team, and it also keeps the formal value of the personal training business low.
4. Build a strong and person-independent team. Because personal training is highly person-dependent, the head of the company must continuously search for good colleagues and then train and coach them.

The exit strategy mostly means that personal training is approached professionally. A personal trainer deals with the same principles that every other business does.

Presentation and Qualifications in Personal Training

A personal trainer should convey a large quantity of characteristics that ensure the client experiences enough value and continues to follow personal training sessions for a longer period of time. The following list provides a short overview:

1. *Professionalism.* It is self-evident that a fitness instructor is professional. However more is demanded of a personal trainer in the area of professional attitude, communication, motivation and follow-up with clients. Generally speaking personal trainers must adopt a more proactive attitude. They must take the lead in coaching clients in every detail of the exercise programme. Nothing is left to chance.

2. *Knowledge and experience.* Personal trainers increase their knowledge in different ways: by following trainings and courses, using systems and reading books and journals. Personal trainers apply the information they read immediately. Another way of learning is by observing professional personal trainers and adopting their

techniques, adjusting them to the personal trainer's own method and philosophy.

3. *Marketing, promotion and sales.* Successful personal trainers are empathic. They promote themselves tactically and dress professionally. Personal trainers use instruments such as personal training promo-boards, business cards and referral cards that look great and a website with testimonials, a strategy where entrepreneurs let someone else tell about their success. Personal trainers also master sales techniques that fit the field of personal training (aimed at the long term) and they regularly review these processes in order to improve.

4. *Integrity and behavioural code.* Professionals such as personal trainers strictly keep to certain behavioural codes and maintain their integrity. This means that they handle information from and about clients carefully and confidentially and practise ethics in matters such as sexuality and etiquette. For more details please see the European Register of Exercise Professionals Code of Ethical Practice, published in *EuropeActive's Foundations for Exercise Professionals* (table 1.5; Rieger et al. 2015).

Table 1.5   The EuropeActive Code of Ethical Practice

'Exercise professionals will be respectful of their customers and of their rights as individuals.'
Compliance with this principle requires personal trainers to maintain a standard of professional conduct appropriate to their dealings with all client groups and to responsibly demonstrate the following:
Respect for individual difference and diversity
Good practice in challenging discrimination and unfairness
Discretion in dealing with confidential client disclosure
'Exercise professionals will nurture healthy relationships with their clients and other health professionals.'
Compliance with this principle requires personal trainers to develop and maintain a relationship with clients based on openness, honesty, mutual trust and respect, and to responsibly demonstrate the following:
The ability to prioritise the client's needs and promote the client's welfare and best interests first when planning an appropriate training programme
Clarity in all forms of communication with clients, professional colleagues and medical practitioners, ensuring honesty, accuracy and co-operation when seeking agreements and avoiding misrepresentation or any conflict of interest arising between the client's need and the personal trainer's professional obligations
Integrity as an exercise professional and recognition of the position of trust dictated by that role, ensuring avoidance of any inappropriate behaviour in all client relationships

(continued)

Table 1.5   *(continued)*

'Exercise professionals will demonstrate and promote a clean and responsible lifestyle and conduct.'

Compliance with this principle requires personal trainers to employ proper personal behaviour at all times and to responsibly demonstrate the following:

The high standards of professional conduct appropriate to their dealings with all their client groups that reflect the particular image and expectations relevant to the role of the personal trainer working in the fitness industry, including never smoking, drinking alcohol or taking recreational drugs before or whilst instructing

That they never advocate or condone the use of prohibited drugs or other banned performance-enhancing substances

An understanding of their legal responsibilities and accountability when dealing with the public and honesty and accuracy in substantiating their claims of authenticity when promoting their services in the public domain

A responsible attitude to the care and safety of client participants within the training environment and in planned activities, ensuring that both are appropriate to the needs of the clients

Provision of adequate and appropriate liability and indemnity insurance at all times to protect their clients and prevent any legal liability from arising

An absolute duty of care to be aware of their working environment and to deal with all reasonably foreseeable accidents and emergencies, as well as to protect themselves, their colleagues and clients

'Exercise professionals will seek to adopt the highest level of professional standards in their work and the development of their career.'

Compliance with this principle requires personal trainers to commit to the attainment of appropriate qualifications and ongoing training:

Actively seek to update knowledge and improve their professional skills in order to maintain a quality standard of service, reflecting on their own practice, identifying development needs and undertaking relevant development activities

Accept responsibility and be accountable for professional decisions or actions, welcoming evaluation of their work and recognising the need when appropriate to refer clients to another professional specialist

Maintain their own effectiveness and confine themselves to practising those activities for which their training and competence is recognised by the Register

Marketing and Sales

When it comes to marketing and sales, personal trainers must be familiar with their own personality. Up to a certain degree, a personality can be matched with a certain client. Personal trainers must stay true to themselves. The style of a personal trainer often attracts a specific target group. There are roughly three different types of personal trainers:

1. *The drill sergeant.* When the style of a personal trainer resembles that of a military instructor (the firm approach), this usually attracts well-trained, very fanatic athletes.

2. *The cheerleader.* Personal trainers who motivate with praise ('You can do it! Woo-hoo!') attract a different type of clients from those who like a firm approach.

3. *The teacher/coach.* Personal trainers who are naturally patient and take the time to answer their clients' questions are typical teachers. They are often good with children and adults who have never trained before.

Some clients want a personal trainer who encourages them during exercise. Others prefer a true drill sergeant. With some imagination, other profiles or combinations can be conceived. However the core message is that the specific individuality of the personal trainer should be reflected in their marketing and sales approach.

Personal trainers use various tools to recruit clients. Business cards and mouth-to-mouth advertising prove to be the most common and important tools, according to a study by Horn (2011). Flyers are barely utilised by personal trainers. Personal trainers use the following strategies to differentiate themselves from others: qualifications or education, image, quality labels, versatile offers and high pricing strategies. Personal trainers point to a few pitfalls in the practical application of their profession: price dumps (actions) by chains they work for, price dumps by colleagues and low familiarity with personal trainers and image (potential clients get the wrong idea about what personal training is). Little research has been done on the degree to which consumers understand personal training and their image of personal training. Personal trainers name the following factors as the most important characteristics for personal trainers (in order of most to least often mentioned): social competence, sympathetic look, professionalism, communication skills and leading by example (Horn 2011).

With regard to sales opportunities, personal trainers have three important possibilities. These are primarily the clients in their direct environment, such as members in a fitness club. In a club situation, new clients also arrive at point of sale via purchase. Finally, the personal trainer gets leads by employing the marketing tools previously mentioned. Naturally, there are many special applications for these three main strategies, for instance, through social media and other Internet tools. Personal trainers in fitness clubs often use strategic consulting. Step one in this method is to make informal contact with the client (member interaction). This contact can start with a short meet-and-greet, with general questions like 'How are you doing?' or 'Can I give you some suggestions on your training programme?' The personal trainer will record the number of such contacts. They may come into contact with a certain client multiple times before moving on to step two: making an appointment for a consultation. During this 20- to 30-minute consultation, the personal trainer gives free training and nutrition advice. Again the personal trainer records the number of consultations given and the conversions of member interactions to consultations. Following the consultation the personal trainer gives a presentation of their services.

Both the sales and service processes begin with the personal trainer asking questions, listening and then continuing to ask questions. It is not easy to ask the client meaningful questions that yield information about their different motivations and goals. To ask clients the right questions, personal trainers must be knowledgeable about different types of questions and get involved with the client they are speaking to. The following list distinguishes two types of questions:

1. Open versus closed
   Open questions ('What is important to you within a training programme?')
   Closed questions: can be answered with a yes or no response ('Do you want to lose weight?')
2. Informative, evaluative and personal
   Informative questions ('How many times a week would you like to exercise?')
   Evaluative questions ('Why have you quit fitness before?')
   Personal questions ('Why is losing weight so important to you?')

A client-oriented conversation starts with a few informative and closed questions in the first minute. It is okay to begin with a question where the client is inclined to give a short answer. Because these questions generally do not provide a lot of information, personal trainers should quickly follow up with open and evaluative questions, or those that cannot be answered with a quick yes or no. These sorts of questions challenge the client to tell more.

It is not wise to ask a potential client too many evaluative questions at the start. This can give clients the feeling that they are being interrogated. Be careful with personal questions as well. Personal trainers must establish good rapport with the client before asking a personal question. Personal questions about, for instance, the income of the client should be avoided. Table 1.6 provides guidance on possible questions.

In a conversation with clients personal trainers mostly ask open questions of an evaluative nature. The client's answer will bring up new follow-up questions. To be able to ask a good follow-up question, the personal trainer must listen closely to the client's answer. They should avoid constantly thinking about the next question whilst

Table 1.6   Type of Questions

Question type	Sample questions
Closed/ informative questions	Have you done fitness in the past? How many personal training sessions would you like to do per week? In which personal training programme would you like to participate? Which times suit you best?
Open/evaluative questions	What are your reasons to exercise? Why did you choose personal training? What are your expectations with regard to your training results?
Open/personal questions	Why is losing weight so important to you? How does it feel now that you have lost 10 kilos?

clients are speaking. The following list provides a sample question strategy for personal trainers collecting information from clients:

- Ask an open starting question and invite the client to give an extensive answer, in which they give their own opinion.
- Listen carefully and distinguish various aspects of the client's answer, for example, a client says that he stopped doing fitness in the past because of an injury.
- Remember the word *injury* and ask a follow-up question on the basis of this word when the client is done speaking. When the client gives an extensive answer, you may need to remember several aspects of their response.
- Follow up on the most important aspect that you can distinguish from the client's answer (see example of *injury*).
- Continue to ask questions in this way for some time.

Personal trainers must be able to make a needs analysis after an interview of approximately 20 to 30 minutes (table 1.7). Make use of the sample questions in the following table if necessary.

Personal trainers cannot assume that they are capable of precisely estimating the client's motives or needs. A good needs analysis has to be made. In the conversation with a client, personal trainers should ask the previously mentioned questions from top to bottom and add a few more. They should never ask directly about an exercise form (activity) that a client might want to do. It is essential to win the client's trust step by step. Only then will their underlying motives become clear, such as uncertainty about their body shape. On the basis of the client's motives, goals and motivation, the personal trainer can create a customised programme that best matches the client's needs.

The interaction between personal trainers and their clients primarily occurs during the sessions. These involve intensive contact,

Table 1.7 Phases of a Needs Analysis

Category	Sample questions
Cause	How did you hear about us? What is your reason for hiring a personal trainer?
History	Have you done fitness before or exercised in general? Which sports have you done? Are there physical problems we need to take into consideration?
Motives	What are your main reasons for exercising? What motivations do you have for exercising?
Goals	What do you want to achieve? When would you like to achieve your goals?
Motivation	Which requirements should a fitness programme meet? What do you think you will like best? What appeals to you least?
Activities	Which form of training appeals most to you? Why? What is the current status of your nutrition programme? When would you like to start: this week or next week?

especially during one-to-one sessions. However contact with clients also takes place before and after sessions. Contact with clients occurs in the following ways:

- Face to face
- Telephone
- Internet (including e-mail and social media such as Twitter)
- Postcards

In addition to these four channels of contact, there are three types of contacts with clients:

- Evaluative: social or relating to content
- Advising: on a physical or mental level
- Motivational: focus on perseverance, fun

In evaluative contact, personal trainers look back on their previous session or look ahead to the next session. This can be social, but will in many cases also relate to the content of the programme. This often changes into an advising contact: The client gets new tips, or is reminded of existing guidelines. The contact often also has a motivational element. The client is stimulated to continue.

Contact Planning

From the combination of channels of contact and content of contacts, the personal trainer can create a basic schematic plan. In the best-case scenario, they enter this plan in an online CRM system, so they never miss an important contact. Please note: This plan should certainly not be followed too strictly. It remains a *personal* training experience for the client; therefore flexibility and client feelings are very important. However the plan does offer guidance and consistency.

Conclusion

This chapter discusses the framework for the profession of personal training. Personal training in Europe appears to be growing rapidly, but because research is limited, it is currently difficult to picture an objective status quo. Basic information is lacking on the amount of personal trainers, clients of personal training and quality. Positive developments include the intent of the European Register of Exercise Professionals to improve the quality of this sector by providing minimum levels of requirements. When focusing on building the future of personal training, personal trainers should keep the end-user in mind in all situations. How can they win and keep the client's trust? That should be the main question that drives all personal training development. To build trust, workers in this sector must create quality and transparency. But at the same time, they must also maintain the diversity and entrepreneurship that have started this profession! This is a fantastic challenge for the future of the fitness sector.

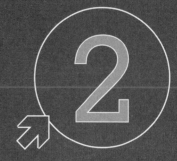

Planning a Personal Training Session

Davide Filingeri

Thomas Rieger

Personal training is a very individual service. It comes quite close to a medical treatment. Therefore every personal training session requires thorough planning. The present chapter provides a comprehensive overview about the most important aspects for personal trainers to master in order to be well prepared and client-oriented in sessions. Based on the principles and characteristics of personal training, this chapter covers implications for the following pivotal areas: session planning to prevent deficient service situations, specific planning instructions for different environments and how personal trainers can successfully apply a proactive role in the adaptation process towards a solid goal achievement, especially when first working with a client. The chapter should primarily be read in conjunction with chapter 3 as well as with selected chapters from the first two books in this series.

Principles and Characteristics of Personal Training

Personal training is a unique type of physical activity instruction characterised by the one-to-one relationship between the personal trainer and the client. This relationship represents the consequence of a client's definite personal choice: the will to reach a specific goal (e.g., wellness, fitness, health) through a specifically designed and carefully supervised training plan. Although many fitness programmes such as aerobics, Pilates or resistance training can lead to the satisfaction of several personal needs (e.g., fun, well-being, socialisation), only a personal training programme assures a structured and individualised exercise intervention focused on critical factors such as the personal aims of the client, the feasibility of these aims and the internal and external motivations (Kraemer and Ratamess 2004). A close relationship with clients allows personal trainers to collect a wide variety of feedback, which they can then use to reshape the exercise programme according to their clients' difficulties and progresses. As a result, when compared to class activities, the individualised intervention of a personal training programme usually translates into an increased likelihood of achieving the goal set (Ratamess et al. 2008; Olney et al. 2006; Mazzetti et al. 2000). Thus personal training can be understood as a fitness service that goes one step farther than the conventional services provided in gyms and other training centres. The latter, especially in Europe, involves one instructor supervising the clients training on the gym floor. Ideally the instructor walks around and tries to make contact with all the clients present in order to meet the minimum requirements of a sufficient fitness service, such as motivating and building rapport.

Against the background of relevant social developments like diversity of lifestyles and individualised demand, the future market for personal training looks promising. People increasingly tend to want customised products and services, and the sporting goods manufacturers that dominate the market have responded to this desire by offering customised lines of their different product segments. People also strive to distinguish themselves, and are willing to pay more to be addressed individually. This tendency seems to be even more relevant in exercise and fitness businesses than in other markets. This is due to the characteristics of the related services that are explained in some chapters of the first two books of this series (see Rieger 2015a; 2015b). Instead of being supervised superficially like in a regular gym setting, clients want to be understood as individuals. They know that an exercise service can be successful only if the programme is based on personal information and grounded in a very intimate relationship. This relationship is so intimate because the personal trainer and client have to engage with each other.

We could better understand the distinction between a fitness instructor and a personal trainer by comparing these differences in roles to those of a lifeguard and a swimming instructor. As mentioned earlier fitness instructors serve as a sort of group supervisor on the gym floor, moving around and making contact with clients. It is clear that the quality of service in a gym setting cannot be the same as in a personal training session. The likelihood of neglecting the most important part of supervision in a gym setting, namely to support clients in achieving their goals, is very high due to the superficial nature of the exchange between clients and the fitness instructor. In this situation instructors primarily tend to correct movements to help clients avoid injuries, for example, correcting bad posture, which is essential, but not expedient in terms of getting stronger or leaner or feeling better. With regard to the lack of time and the high number of clients, who very often want to be served simultaneously, the role of fitness instructors can be interpreted as similar to that of the lifeguard: They mainly prevent damage rather than furthering training success. Personal trainers work under better conditions. They perform like swimming instructors, building a close relationship with the client. They know important information about their clients, such as their personalities. These are all relevant prerequisites in order to help clients improve. Moreover, personal trainers have a detailed perspective on the training process, and can accordingly plan the activities appropriately.

Planning Activities

First and foremost, all planning activities have to be based on the wishes and preferences of the client. With regard to satisfaction achievement, the personal trainer needs to make assiduous efforts in terms of client orientation. The client determines where and when the service takes place, whether indoors or outdoors, in the morning, afternoon or evening. It is the personal trainer's responsibility to learn the client's preferences and develop the best programme and timetable possible in order to help the client achieve the determined goals. The personal trainer therefore needs to listen very carefully and apply instinctive feeling to find the optimal balance between meeting the client's wishes and achieving the best outcome possible. Building rapport is key here because it helps the client share the necessary information (Rieger 2015a). In planning a personal training programme personal trainers must be able to design a timetable of sessions in which each training unit contributes *micro goals* to the achievement of a *macro goal* (Kraemer et al. 2009; table 2.1).

The timetable should be based on the clear understanding of the client's needs and should be both accurately structured and adaptable. The personal trainer's ability to prescribe and manage the activities will help them balance this apparent contrast between the rigidity and flexibility that such an intervention requires. For

Table 2.1 How to Reach a Macro Goal Through Step-by-Step Micro Goals

Level	Macro goal	Micro goal 1	Micro goal 2	Micro goal 3	Micro goal 4
Beginner	Running: 25 min	Running: 10 min, low intensity	Running: 15 min, low intensity	Running: 15 min, moderate intensity	Running: 20 min, moderate intensity
Intermediate	Push-ups: 10 reps	Knee push-up: 10 reps	Hand step push-up: 5 reps	Push-up: 5 reps	Push-up: 8 reps
Advanced	Pull-ups: 10 reps	Lat machine: 10 reps 50% body weight	Lat machine: 8 reps 100% body weight	Rubber band assisted pull-up: 10 reps	Pull-up: 5 reps

instance, the combination of supervised and unsupervised activities is often a winning choice for promoting behavioural changes leading to healthy lifestyles. The supervised sessions aim to deliver the training intervention in an encouraging environment, where the presence of the personal trainer supports the client in a step-by-step progression. During these sessions, the personal trainer provides a real time control of the practice, accurate information on the aims of the exercises and an individualised motivational support (Donnelly et al. 2009).

Unsupervised sessions (e.g., home-based exercises, jogging, cycling or swimming) also contribute significantly to the organisation of the timetable. These sessions have the potential to create and build up the client's sense of autonomy and self-confidence. Unsupervised sessions are the result of clear and simple prescriptions, and can complement the main workout programme (table 2.2).

Since the personal trainer will be absent during unsupervised activities, they should be introduced when the client has reached a sufficient level of practice. This *threshold* is set by the personal trainer in evaluating the achievement of specific micro goals, such as correct exercise technique, client perception of their own limits and self-management of fatigue and stress (Garber et al. 2011). The personal trainer should always aim for a comfortable balance between supervised and unsupervised sessions. One important aspect in this regard is trust, which is created through rapport building (see Rieger 2015a). The personal trainer must rely on clients' feedback about how they performed in unsupervised sessions.

As mentioned previously personal training is a very individualised exercise service. Hence every session should be considered unique, and requires special preparation (Kieß 2012). Each day is different,

Table 2.2   Guidelines for Unsupervised Training Units (TU) Within a Weekly Training Programme

TU 1	TU 2	TU 3	TU 4
Supervised	Unsupervised	Supervised	Unsupervised
N/A	**Aim:** 20 min running	N/A	**Aim:** 25 min cycling
	Guidelines		**Guidelines**
	Warm-up Parking the car 10 min walking distance away from the running area and walking there + 5 min stretching		Warm-up Walking up and down stairs (at least 3 floors) × 2 + 5 min stretching
	Running 5 min: 40–50% HRmax* 5 min: 50–60% HRmax 5 min: 60–70% HRmax 5 min: 40–50% HRmax		Cycling 5 min: 40–50% HRmax 5 min: 70–80% HRmax 5 min: 40–50% HRmax 5 min: 70–80% HRmax 5 min: 40–50% HRmax
	Cool-down Walking to the car + 5 min stretching		Cool-down Walking 5 min + 5 min stretching

*HRmax = Heart Rate Maximum

for the personal trainer as well as for the client. The following example gives an impression about how an individual approach can be implemented into the everyday routine. Assuming that the personal trainer has scheduled their next client session at 4 p.m. in the gym, they must start the preparation for the session around 30 minutes in advance in order to cover the following steps:

1. If this is the first appointment of the day, the personal trainer should commence their preparation at home by checking their personal look, including shaving, hairstyle and appropriateness and cleanliness of clothing.

2. The personal trainer should gather all documents required for the appointment: current training plan, papers from previous training assessments (mood of client, level of performance, motivation), macro and micro goal sheets and the template for the upcoming training assessment. They should also thoroughly check any apps or other electronic tools being used for training documentation.

After arriving at the gym, the personal trainer should continue with the following steps:

1. Gathering and checking functionality of small tools like heart rate monitor, scale, writing utensils
2. Checking availability, functionality and cleanliness of training equipment like machines and free weights. If possible, the equipment should be placed in the right order, so that interruptions are minimised.
3. Mentally focusing on the upcoming appointment by going through all possible eventualities that could occur
4. Finally, shifting into rapport mode. This means that the personal trainer should sharpen concentration and mentally go through the pivotal elements of building rapport before meeting the client (see Rieger 2015a).

All these preparatory steps should be implemented as a mandatory routine for the personal trainer because they are linked to an important part of service quality management, potential quality (see Rieger 2015b). The included potentials define the quality basis for the service itself, which is called *process quality*, and for the expected outcomes (e.g., well-being, satisfaction). Neglecting the aforementioned preparatory aspects increases the likelihood of obtaining suboptimal results for the process and the outcomes. It does not matter where the personal training session takes place (in the gym, in the forest or a park), preparation is always pivotal. The following section differentiates between the two most important environments for personal training sessions, the indoor and the outdoor setting.

Planning and Improvising Effective Activities for Different Environments

Traditionally fitness activities are performed in well-furnished fitness centres. Despite this a personal trainer should be able to organise indoor and outdoor activities by optimising the use of any resource or device. Any part of the environment in which the activity is performed can become part of the training session. If an unexpected occurrence (e.g., sudden unavailability of resources like machines or free weights) arises, the personal trainer should be ready to improvise the content of the session and provide appropriate alternatives that still meet the requirements for that specific session (i.e., certain training goals) whilst maintaining a pleasant experience for the client. Note that improvising a session with alternative resources can also represent a moment of discovery and challenge for the client. Because these could contribute to maintaining high levels of interest and involvement with the programme, according to the client's profile, *improvised sessions* might be therefore planned in advance by the personal trainer as part of the programme. This of course depends on the personality and wishes of the client, but alternating environments can usually support motivation and compliance to the prescribed overall programme (Klein 1997).

As mentioned before the most obvious distinction of environments is between indoor and outdoor. In terms of preparation, planning and improvising of the sessions, personal trainers should consider several specifics as well as eventualities and different scenarios.

Indoor

If the personal trainer delivers the session in their private gym with their own equipment and schedule, the likelihood of interrupting events is low. In a regular gym, where clients move in and out, the situation is different. The most critical point in this regard is the availability of training machines. For example, if there is only one horizontal leg press available in the gym and the session is sched-uled for 6 p.m. (i.e., training rush hour), the personal trainer should probably find equipment alternatives such as other variations on the leg press or squat machines. Moreover the personal trainer should be aware of any disturbing noise levels during this time of the day. Thus in sessions during busy times at the gym, the personal trainer should avoid presenting new or demanding exercise instructions. Another problematic situation that could occur when training in the gym involves other gym customers approaching the personal trainer and client. Very often personal trainers work for the gym in different functions like fitness or group instructors. Gym members who know the personal trainer from other gym activities might approach the trainer during one-to-one sessions with a paying client. This is a tricky situation. On the one hand the personal trainer wants to give his full attention to the paying client; on the other hand he cannot snub the other customer, since the customer may not be able to assess the situation correctly. It is a difficult balance. Whenever possible, personal trainers should try to bypass these situations in advance. Avoiding rush hours in the morning and afternoon is highly recommended. All these aspects should be taken into consideration.

Outdoor

Outdoor settings can be very motivating for clients, and can help members who primarily prefer the classical gym training approach overcome boredom. For clients who spend most of their day at a desk or in enclosed areas, the personal trainer should recommend increasing physical activity and spending more time outside to enjoy nature and fresh air in calm and peaceful surroundings. Clients have an easier time forgetting about their daily job routines when outdoors. Small or compact training devices can add a lot of variety to outdoor personal training.

As with indoor sessions, personal trainers must practise proper planning, including anticipating worst-case scenarios. The personal trainer must be aware that uncontrollable factors can affect the service quality or can even lead to cancellation of the session. The first and foremost factor in this regard is weather conditions. If the personal trainer is located in the temperate climate zone, the best periods throughout the year are between April and June and from the end of August until late October, when temperatures are very comfortable. July and August can also be feasible as long as temperatures are not too high. If clients are willing to do sessions outdoors, these pleasant months should be prioritised. Outdoor training is very variable. The session can be performed in one place, can be set up as a running track with different stations, or simply include a running workout. In case of choosing one of the track options, the personal trainer needs to check several factors, such as track profile (including climbs and drops), possible traffic issues, ground profile (forest soil, asphalt) and humidity. Hence, they also should provide knowledgeable tips about appropriate shoes for the weather conditions. If sessions take place in late fall or winter, especially during morning or evening hours, darkness can be an issue. Personal trainers must check pathways and routes for light conditions. If a client prefers training at these times of day, the personal trainer should seriously think about offering special lighting systems, although in this case, they must also remember to check the batteries, reliability of the system and so on. In addition to activities based on running, personal trainers can consider other functional and strength training activities like biking or swimming. Because these activities are very complicated in terms of preparation (e.g., swimming techniques, access to a pool, biking equipment, traffic issues), and should therefore play only a minor role in the arsenal of the personal trainer's activities for cardiorespiratory exercise, this chapter does not elaborate on them further (please see Hines 2008 and Sovndal 2013 for more information).

For the concrete delivery of sessions in different environments and their related advantages and disadvantages, please see chapter 3.

Planning Activities to Support the Individual Adaptation Process

The personal trainer's role in leading a client to actively participate in a training programme is essential (Saetre et al. 2011). Their aim should be to promote adherence to healthy lifestyle models by offering active support. Individualised support represents a critical determinant of the client's success, and it is fundamental in the adaptation process for each client (Kuhr et al. 2011), particularly at the beginning of the training relationship. In these early stages the risk of dropout is indeed high. Several reasons can contribute to this behaviour: For example, high expectations of immediate results can lead to disappointing outcomes, thus inducing a lack of motivation in completing the programme. As such, the personal trainer should create environmental conditions that make the client feel self-confident as well as become aware that outcomes will result from a medium- to long-term practice, according to the physiological and psychological adaptation processes (table 2.3).

The achievement of the client's final goals will result from an informed and structured practice. This will progressively give clients the awareness that they are *active players* rather than *passive receivers* of the adaption process (Van Asselt et al. 2011). Each client presents individual needs, and as such personal trainers should create a unique profile for clients that they can track. Focusing on and adapting to these aspects, from time to time, allows the personal trainer to establish a confident and empathy-based relationship that leads, through the training programme, to a deeply rooted behavioural change in the client's lifestyle.

In order to maximise the outcomes of each individual adaptation process, namely to achieve visible and remarkable physical and

Table 2.3   Managing Factors Contributing to Training Program Dropout

Reason	How to prevent the problem	How to deal with the problem
High expectations of immediate results	Inform clients in a clear and easy way about the time requirements of the general physiological adaptations of the human body	Analyse the client's personal profile and behaviour
	Inform clients about the training plan and when to expect the first results	Give simple examples of adaptive processes
Disappointed expectations	Monitor outcomes of training sessions	Evaluate the predictability and the unpredictability of the causes responsible for the failure
	Monitor client's feedback on training status	Plan new activities to reduce the error percentage
Lack of motivation	Plan quantifiable micro goals	Critically analyse the client's expectations
	Introduce a variety of training experiences	Critically analyse the achieved results

mental improvements accompanied by client satisfaction, personal trainers must plan each session thoroughly in order to stick to the determined pathway towards the micro and macro goals. Planning in this regard means to reflect every session against the defined goal system. This is not about the preparation of training equipment or of other props, which are undoubtedly important (see earlier passages in this chapter); rather this is a question of maintaining the overview of the overall framework. Between training sessions, the personal trainer should invest at least 15 minutes to review the client's past workouts. Therefore personal trainers must maintain robust training documentation, both paper based and technology based.

Documentation facilitates goal achievement by allowing personal trainers to constantly track the necessary physical, mental and performance parameters such as weights, repetitions, heart rate under stress, mood and body weight. They can easily monitor deficits in order to provide any needed intervention immediately. Thus every session is grounded in current data. The selection of assessed parameters of course depends on the client's goals. This approach leads to a dynamic training relation between the personal trainer and client that goes beyond the more-or-less static training plan developed in the beginning. Moreover it fulfils another important role. Very detailed documentation of the training process allows the personal trainer to visualise step-by-step improvements for the client. From a motivation standpoint this is very crucial because the possibility that clients will quit is very high, especially in the beginning of a training process (Middelkamp and Rieger 2013). Hence proper planning of training sessions in terms of goals can positively affect client motivation.

Conclusion

When it comes to success in fitness, performance or well-being, every session and every surrounding aspect must be optimised. Each personal training session, no matter in which environment it takes place, requires thorough planning. First personal trainers must care for their personal appearance, sharpen their concentration before the session and gather all necessary devices, equipment and papers. The key motto here is 'Be ready.' Finalising the checklist is a prerequisite for delivering a first-class service. Second the personal trainer is responsible for the client's level of goal achievement. In this context planning also comes into play. Planning includes goal monitoring that is both permanent and sustainable, where the personal trainer emphasises the need for visualising the attainment of subgoals. The client will likely experience stronger motivation if they realise that they are moving forward towards the main goal step by step, session by session. Thus planning is of vital importance for the client and the personal trainer. Better outcomes due to steady motivation lead to satisfied clients and, in the end, to a more successful business for the personal trainer.

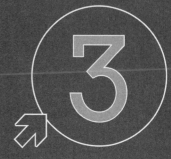

Delivering a Personal Training Session

Nuno Pimenta

The main role of a personal trainer is to promote healthy lifestyles by helping clients change unhealthy behaviours and adopt proper exercise and healthy diets, and they should take this into account in all their tasks. This chapter focuses on delivering an exercise session to a client and on what it involves. Before starting an exercise programme the personal trainer must assess the client's health status, lifestyle, health-related and skill-related fitness and primary goals. Based on all the data gathered from the client the personal trainer can then develop an individualised exercise programme. A training session may be considered as a small unit of an exercise program.

Remember that a personal training session is not a homogenous activity, with all components equal from beginning to end. The training session is usually divided in several parts. The specific components that should be included in a personal training session depend on the client's goals, needs and expectations. The most common and important components of an exercise session include the warm-up, a conditioning phase, the cool-down and stretching (Brooks 2004; Riebe 2013a). Each of these components has its own characteristics and particular purposes. The warm-up helps the client make a safe transition from rest to exercise, and the conditioning phase leads the client to achieve their training goals. The cool-down should assure a safe return from exercise back to the resting state, followed by stretching, which is intended to reduce muscle tension and postexercise muscle soreness as well as maintain range of motion (ROM) in the joints. The personal trainer must follow the client throughout the whole session, and should be proficient in all exercise session components such as monitoring and adjusting exercise, maintaining good communication, motivating the clients and taking advantage of different training environments and taking advantage also of technology to promote frequent and good communication with the client.

Monitoring and Adjusting Exercise

In the design of an exercise programme, the personal trainer needs to make decisions about the characteristics of the exercise, often called *exercise prescription components*, based on what will best address the client's goals and needs. Next the personal trainer needs to implement and monitor such a programme. Once the plan has been put into practice, the personal trainer may realise that the decisions made when preparing the exercise programme are not appropriate for the client. In that case the personal trainer must identify the need for technical intervention (adjustments) to make the programme better suited to the client. Personal trainers can adjust the exercise prescription components themselves, or other aspects related to exercise execution and safety.

Exercise Prescription Components

Exercise prescription usually follows the FITT-VP principle (Riebe 2013a), which stands for frequency (how often), intensity (how hard), time (how long) and type (what kind) of exercise, plus the exercise volume (frequency × intensity × time) and progression. Personal trainers must tailor these exercise prescription components well when planning sessions so that the client will comply with the programme and achieve the desired goals.

The need for adjustments may occur with virtually any exercise prescription component. Table 3.1 presents some common situations that can occur (although the solutions for any specific situation may depend greatly on the characteristics of the client and their desired goals).

Execution of the Exercises

One of the most important interventions is related to how an exercise is performed. The personal trainer must be able to intervene to help the client demonstrate safe and effective exercise technique.

Table 3.1 Common Exercise Situations Requiring Adjustments

Situation (Description of the circumstances requiring adjustments)	Problem (Identification of the exercise prescription component that needs adjustment)	Solution (Example of an adjustment made to refine exercise for the client)
The client shows evident signs of fatigue, and is struggling to comply with the exercise (e.g., the client cannot speak more than two words in a row whilst running at the determined speed, and is struggling to keep up with the exercise).	The intensity is too high for the client (probably well above the lactate threshold, in the case of cardiorespiratory exercise), and they will not be able to keep up with the exercise as prescribed.	The personal trainer needs to reduce one of the two mechanical variables of intensity (speed [km/h] or incline [%]) in order to bring the intensity under the lactate threshold so that the client can perform the exercise continuously. An alternative solution, if the client is at a more advanced stage, is to design an interval training programme so that the client can reach the initially determined intensity of exercise with rest periods in between.
The client consistently finishes the exercises before the duration predetermined in the exercise programme.	One of three problem may be commonly diagnosed: 1. Intensity is too high. 2. Duration is too long. 3. The client lacks will or motivation.	1. The intensity (either speed or resistance in the case of cardiorespiratory exercise; the load in the case of strength training, and so on) may be reduced. 2. The duration (kilometres or minutes in the case of cardiorespiratory exercise; number of repetitions or time in the case of strength training, and so on) may be reduced. 3. Sometimes the personal trainer needs only to communicate with the client to raise their motivation (models and theories are discussed in another section of this chapter).
The client keeps missing exercise sessions.	The frequency of exercise is not appropriate for the client's needs.	Exercise frequency needs to be adjusted to the client's constraints and availability, and not only to the client's goals. The personal trainer should also evaluate whether the goals are realistic and set step-by-step partial goals that the client can achieve in the short term (e.g., including two sessions of exercise every week in a row for a month).

(continued)

Table 3.1 *(continued)*

Situation (Description of the circumstances requiring adjustments)	Problem (Identification of the exercise prescription component that needs adjustment)	Solution (Example of an adjustment made to refine exercise for the client)
The client feels abnormally fatigued in a specific exercise, even though they are performing at the same relative intensity as another exercise (e.g., unsuccessfully attempting an exercise at the same 80% of HR reserve that they did successfully on the treadmill). The client may also seem particularly demotivated and bored in a specific exercise.	The type or mode of exercise may be influencing the client's response to the exercise programme.	The personal trainer should assess the client's tastes and habits regarding exercise. A type of exercise that the client is unaccustomed to may lead to early fatigue, as compared to a familiar exercise form. On such exercises the client should perform at lower intensities to start and then progress step by step over a couple of weeks until reaching the desired intensity. Similarly forms of exercise that the client is not particularly fond of may have a detrimental effect on the exercise programme. Personal trainers should identify and fix such situations early in the programme, finding a type of exercise that the client is more comfortable or happy with.
The client completes the exercise session with very little effort.	The exercise programme is no longer meeting the overload principle of training.	It is now time to progress the exercise programme. The client needs to face a higher physiological/mechanical challenge in order to keep making the adaptations that will ultimately lead them to their exercise goals.

Interventions include good instruction, demonstration and explanation of the critical components of each exercise, and proficiency in identifying the client's execution errors, correcting those mistakes in execution and adjusting exercises when needed.

A good *instruction* is usually a short communication where the personal trainer focuses on the most important aspects of the exercise that will guarantee that the client can start the exercise without serious errors, particularly those that could threaten their safety. Many times this includes a *demonstration* of the exercise by the personal trainer so that the client will have a visual image of what is intended. The content (information) of the instruction and the way of saying it (rehearsal effect) can be practised so that the personal trainer will come across as secure, experienced and proficient and will effectively convey the message.

The personal trainer must be able to identify and correct any exercise execution errors, bad posture or mistakes that the client may engage in right when they occur. Both capacities are crucial. Identifying errors is probably the hardest skill, especially for novice personal trainers, but it becomes easier with experience. Correcting errors properly, giving appropriate feedback and using the right correction techniques to solve the problem are also very important.

Sometimes to make an exercise appropriate for a particular client the personal trainer must adjust the exercise. This includes changing exercise prescription components, modifying exercises and sometimes substituting one exercise for another.

Table 3.2 describes different types of interventions. These may include simple feedback or more intensive interventions, such as asking the client to stop the exercise so that the personal trainer can give a demonstration or additional explanation. Personal trainers should carefully consider the type of intervention needed for a given situation before making it. If the personal trainer gives only feedback, the client may receive this as a normal intervention. But if the personal trainer asks the client to stop the exercise, they may perceive this as failure, which will probably make them feel bad about the training session. It is the personal trainer's job to counteract such feelings by using good communication, assuming a pedagogic attitude, explaining to the client what is happening at all times and paying special attention to the motivational aspects of the communication with the client. As a rule personal trainers should interrupt an exercise only when the identified errors relate to safety issues. If the physical integrity of the client is not at stake, most of the times there is no reason to interrupt the exercise.

Safety

Another main task of the personal trainer is to promote the highest safety standards during the preparation of the exercise programme (based on a sound assessment of the client's medical history, lifestyle and fitness) and throughout all training sessions. Exercise does involve some risks, particularly in clients with chronic conditions and when appropriate assessment is not considered and proper exercise prescription guidelines are not followed (CSEP 2010; Thompson 2013). However as a general rule moderate exercise is very safe, and provides health benefits even for sedentary, higher risk populations (Clark et al. 2005).

Clients may encounter two main types of risks related to exercise: orthopaedic risk and metabolic risk. Orthopaedic risk is mainly related to the technical execution of the exercises and postures, and may result in joint and muscle injuries. It can be prevented with a

Table 3.2 Sample Interventions for Client Corrections

Situation (Description of the setting)	Problem (Identification of the problem)	Solution (Description of possible solutions)
The client is continuously performing the cycle ergometer exercise.	The client is struggling a little with the intensity, and their knees are almost touching their elbows.	Ask the client to stop the exercise and push the seat up to increase its height in the cycle ergometer. This will allow a better execution of the exercise and enhanced muscle participation and will hopefully reduce the client's struggle.
The client is trying to execute knee raises in supine position (similar to abdominal crunch but lifting the pelvic waist from the floor instead of the scapular waist).	The client does not understand how to execute the exercise and keeps executing it incorrectly even after a throughout instruction and sound feedback.	Ask the client to execute a different exercise that works the same muscle group but is easier to execute (e.g., change from a knee raise in supine position to a knee raise in a vertical hanging position, supported by the elbows and forearms on a structure or machine, and reducing the number of repetitions). Changing the exercise is the best solution when, for some reason, the client seems to have a mental barrier to understanding critical components of an exercise.
The client is performing continuous cardiorespiratory exercise on an elliptical ergometer.	The client is doing the exercise in bursts with constant stops. It seems like the resistance is too high. The client is trying to make rotational instead of an elliptical movement.	Ask the client to use a different ergometer for the same muscle group and to change from the elliptical ergometer to a treadmill (also a weight-bearing ergometer) or a cycle ergometer (also circular movement with reduced impact). This is the best solution when, for some reason, the client seems to have a mental barrier to understanding critical components of an exercise.
The client is executing a supine full plank, supported by the elbows and forearms on the floor.	The client seems to understand how the exercise is done and tries to execute it well, but struggles to hold a correct position for the prescribed time.	Adjust the exercise by changing from a full plank to a plank with knees on the floor. This will maintain the general aspects and muscle participation of the exercise but will reduce the intensity by reducing the length of the resistance arm, and therefore will make the exercise easier for the client to execute correctly.

good selection of exercises and effective correction of execution errors and bad posture. Metabolic risk is mainly related to exercise intensity and to the client's particular characteristics, including undiagnosed health problems that may lead to abnormal responses to exercise such as sudden drops in blood pressure, myocardial infarction or stroke. Sound guidelines for assessing the client and defining the specific dimension of the metabolic challenge to be imposed can be easily found in publications in the field (ACSM 2013; CSEP 2010).

Metabolic risk can be decreased by assessing the client's response to exercise using available strategies. For example during continuous cardiorespiratory exercise, the personal trainer can use a heart rate monitor to verify if the client is in the predetermined target zone. They can also use the talk test (Persinger et al. 2004), asking the client to speak a few words in a row. If the client has a hard time speaking more than a few words without getting out of breath, the exercise intensity may be too high. In other forms of exercise the personal trainer should maintain good communication with the client to assess whether they feel well and comfortable; for example the rating of perceived exertion (RPE) scale—also called the Borg scale—can be used (Irving et al. 2006; von Leupoldt et al. 2006).

The bottom line is that the personal trainer is responsible for assuring a healthy and safe exercise during all training sessions and workouts, following clients, identifying dangerous situations and intervening accordingly.

Maintaining Good Communication and Motivation

A primary duty of any personal trainer is to establish sound and fruitful communication with the client. A good starting point is to understand that the client is the boss; therefore the personal trainer must have the tools to assure professional, correct, joyful and powerful communication with all clients.

Some personal trainers struggle with barriers for establishing communication with clients in a more informal and unstructured fashion. This happens particularly with novice personal trainers, who are often more focused on communication about the exercise prescription components (Bonelli 2000). With experience communication with the clients may progressively become more influenced by motivational aspects, thereby creating an environment where the clients feel good about the exercise and themselves (Bonelli 2000).

Some personal trainers have difficulty communicating effectively with their clients. To boost communication competence, personal trainers can use insightful strategies and plentiful practice.

Comprehensive strategies may include practising predetermined short phrases that will provide important feedback to a client during a session (e.g., 'I'm very proud of you'; 'Keep your shoulders down'; 'Great job'; 'Please keep your knees aligned with your toes.') in front of a mirror to find the best way to look and sound convincing or, in other words, to find the best way to convey the message.

Besides their own personal characteristics, personal trainers must take the client's characteristics into account. They should be aware of two approaches related to communication. One approach is the learning style or cognitive style, which aims to identify the client's general characteristics and preferences. The second approach is more focused on motivation and long-term behavioural change, and is based on psychological models such as the transtheoretical model or the self-determination model.

The *learning style* theories proposed over the past 30 years may help personal trainers to get in tune with the client (Dunn 1990; Felder and Silverman 1988; Fleming 2001; Gregorc 1979; Kolb 1984). One simple theory is the VARK model (an acronym for visual, aural, reading/writing and kinaesthetic learning styles), originally developed by the New Zealand educator Neil Fleming, which takes exclusively into account a client's characteristics and preferred ways of gathering, organizing and thinking information (Fleming and Mills 1992). The VARK model should be considered an instructional preference model because it is based and organised according to a person's perceptual modes (with the exception of smell and taste; Hawk and Shah 2007). For example, some clients prefer, or are better at, appropriating verbal information (aural). Others do well with visual information, and some may even have a preference for several or all the learning styles. A client's learning style preferences can be easily assessed using specific inventories, scales or questionnaires. For the VARK model, Neil Fleming developed a questionnaire (available online at www.vark-learn.com; Fleming 2001).

After determining a client's learning style preferences, the personal trainer can then convey instruction, information and feedback. Table 3.3 describes the VARK model's learning styles and presents strategies for adapting communication for each learning style so that personal trainers can convey their messages in a way that is easy for clients to receive. Note that, in some cases, one learning style rises above all the others. There is no specific column in table 3.3 for a multimodal learning style profile (e.g., a visual-aural, or a reader/writer-kinaesthetic, or even a visual-aural-reader/writer-kinaesthetic). In those cases, the personal trainer should use mixed strategies from all the columns corresponding to the client's learning style profile. Regardless of the client's learning style profile, the preferences of a client should have a significant effect on the personal trainer's selection of optimal communication strategies.

Sometimes, particularly in the context of personal training, it is not easy to apply such questionnaires or inventories, mainly because the bulk of session time is needed for interventions regarding the client's goals, needs and expectations. Therefore the personal trainer will not have access to the collected data. If that occurs, they should deliver the instruction, information and feedback to the client using multiple approaches so that it is suitable for every learning style. Though this may seem quite demanding for personal trainers, it will help them communicate more effectively and be more successful in their role.

Along with the professional relationship with a client, the personal trainer may subjectively notice the client showing some preferences for a particular learning style. In this case they may intentionally emphasise communication strategies that address that learning style. Table 3.4 presents tips for subjectively identifying clients' learning styles.

Table 3.3   Description of VARK Model Learning Styles and Specific Approaches Regarding Each Profile (Fleming 2001)

	Visual	Aural	Read/Write	Kinaesthetic
Description	Preferences for graphical and symbolic ways of representing information	Preferences for heard information	Preferences for information printed as words	Preferences for information taken from experience and practice
How to intervene	Diagrams, graphs, colours, charts, different fonts, spatial arrangement, designs	Debates, arguments, discussions, conversations, audio recordings, videos with audio, seminars, music	Books, texts, handouts, written feedback, notes, essays, multiple choice tests, bibliographies	Demonstrations, real-life examples, simulated examples, physical activity, role play, working models

Table 3.4   Characteristics of Learning Styles*

Visual	Aural	Read/Write	Kinaesthetic
Speaks rapidly with frequent use of voice inflexions	Speaks rhythmically and rarely uses voice inflexions	Speaks rapidly and may use voice inflexions	Speaks slowly and pauses frequently
Eyes look up or straight ahead to access information	Looks side to side to access information	Eyes look up or straight ahead to access information	Looks down to access information
Influenced most by what they see	Influenced most by what they hear	Influenced most by what they read	Influenced most by what they feel
Frequent use of body gestures	Moderate use of body gestures	May use body gestures frequently	Moves slowly, infrequent use of body gestures

*Based on neurolinguistics and adapted to the VARK model.

The second approach regarding *behavioural theories and models* is also a cornerstone for personal trainers. Several theories and models have been proposed, some focusing particularly on exercise (Riebe 2013b). These models and theories influence the content of the information to be given to a client, unlike the previously described learning theories that influence mostly the way the information is delivered to the client but not its content.

Concepts such as the theory of self-efficacy, the transtheoretical model and the self-determination theory have been advocated as useful for increasing participation in recreational physical activity, and therefore are valuable tools for the personal trainer (Riebe 2013b).

Self-efficacy is the central component of many behavioural theories. It has been defined as the belief in one's capabilities to successfully organise and execute the required actions for a given goal (Ashford et al. 2010). The concept of self-efficacy relies on the postulate that cognitive processes mediate behaviour change, but that cognitive events are induced and altered more readily by the experience of mastery arising from effective performance (Bandura 1977). According to this theoretical framework a personal trainer may promote exercise participation or adherence by increasing the client's awareness or belief that they are capable and proficient in completing the actions proposed by the personal trainer (Ashford et al. 2010).

The *transtheoretical model*, initially proposed by Prochaska and colleagues (1992) to help change addictive behaviours, has been adapted to help the process of adopting exercise behaviours (Hutchison et al. 2009). According to this theory everyone is considered to be in one of five proposed stages of readiness for behavioural changes, described in table 3.5. All clients are presumably in one of the three more advanced stages of readiness for behavioural change: prepara-

Table 3.5   The Transtheoretical Model's Stages of Readiness for Behavioural Changes

Stage	Description
Precontemplation	Not intending to take action in the foreseeable future; most likely unaware that their behaviour is problematic and health threatening
Contemplation	Beginning to recognise that their behaviour is problematic and starting to look at the pros and cons of continued actions
Preparation	Intending to take action in the immediate future; may soon begin taking small steps towards change
Action	Already made specific overt modifications in lifestyle, meeting at least the minimum amount of recommended physical activity
Maintenance	Have been in the action stage for 6 months; working to prevent relapse. This stage can last indefinitely.

Adapted from Spencer et al. 2006.

tion (intending to be regularly active in the next 30 days or already somewhat active but not yet meeting the minimal physical activity recommendations), action (regularly active for fewer than 6 months) or maintenance (regularly active for 6 months or more; Spencer et al. 2006). This is because they have already taken the first step to engage in physical exercise, and are presently clients of a personal trainer.

The information a personal trainer gives to a client in the preparation stage should differ from what they would give a client in the action stage, all of which may differ also from the information suitable for a client in the maintenance stage. Ultimately the personal trainer's goal is to intervene with all clients to help them reach more advanced stages of readiness for behavioural change, preferably the maintenance stage (regularly active for 6 months or more). Table 3.6 presents some examples of intervention based on a client's behavioural change readiness stage.

Another keystone theory is the *self-determination theory* (Riebe 2013b). This theory focuses on one's motivation and distinguishes among demotivation (lack of intention to engage in exercise), extrinsic motivation (engaging in exercise for reasons dissociated from the behaviour itself, e.g., 'I exercise because I want to lose weight.') and intrinsic motivation (exercising for pure joy and satisfaction associated with the behaviour itself, e.g., 'I exercise because I love it!') (Silva et al. 2008). This theory also distinguishes between *self-determined motivation* (when it results from the client's own choice and volition, e.g., 'I decided to participate in exercise and my goal is...') and *controlled motivation* (when it results from pressure from others and not from the client themselves, e.g., 'My doctor told me to start exercising.') (Silva et al. 2008). When clients exercise as a result of a self-determined motivation and associate this habit with enjoyment and satisfaction gained from taking part in that behaviour, they are more likely to sustain it in the long run (Teixeira et al. 2012). In other words, a personal trainer should plan and adapt the exercises and communicate with clients in such a way to transform exercise into an intrinsically enjoyable and satisfactory behaviour.

For more intentional and proficient communication with clients, the personal trainer should practise communication techniques in accordance with the theoretical framework set by effective behavioural theories. This approach may enhance the personal trainer's skills and proficiency in communicating and promoting exercise adherence. Sound introductory publications in the field of behaviour change regarding exercise are widely available (ACSM 2013; Martin 2013; McClanahan 2013; Napolitano 2013).

When a personal trainer and a client (or a small group) are developing a professional relationship, strong two-way communication is

Table 3.6 Sample Interventions for Each Stage of Behavioural Change Readiness

Stage	Intervention
Precontemplation	The personal trainer should talk about the benefits of exercise: 'You should consider increasing your physical activity because it may add years to your life and give more life to your years.' 'Increasing physical activity would increase your quality of life and would probably save you some money at the doctor.'
Contemplation	The personal trainer should subtly give the client strategies for overcoming the initial barriers for adopting exercise: 'You could consider taking the stairs more often instead of the elevator.' 'Park your car two blocks away from your destination.' 'We can start by removing as much as possible of your daily sedentary time: Reducing your sitting and screen time may be helpful.'
Preparation	The personal trainer should subtly introduce strategies for increasing daily physical activity: 'Why don't you look for professional services, like a gym or health club or a personal trainer, so that you can reach optimal levels of physical activity and exercise in your life?' 'You could join a walking group in your neighbourhood.' 'Your best option is to ask for the help of a personal trainer.'
Action	The client is already engaged in physical activity, and the personal trainer's challenge is to keep the client in that path. So the personal trainer should introduce activities that, besides promoting all the intended benefits, are enjoyable for the client. This will help clients incorporate the exercises into their lifestyle in the long run. Ways of introducing the idea include the following: 'Now that you're in good shape you'll have no trouble in fitting your company's football team.' 'Now you can have a better time playing tennis with your neighbours and your sons.' 'I'll teach you the basics so that you can easily get into an aerobic dance or Latin class that you love.'
Maintenance	Now that the client has included physical activity in their lifestyle, the personal trainer's challenge is to help them avoid relapse. Clients get tired of working out sometimes or just struggle in keeping up the physical activity routine, and there are loads of motifs for such (e.g., boring or stagnant exercise routine, divorce or other strong events with profound changes in the client's life attitude towards physical activity, job promotions, having a baby or other events with increased responsibilities and reduced spare time). The personal trainer must be well aware of the barriers to staying physically active that clients may encounter, and should intervene to prevent and help clients overcome all those barriers. When relapse occurs the personal trainer must assess the client's readiness for behavioural change and intervene accordingly.

needed. This requires personal trainers to be proficient at acknowledging what the client says. There is an old saying 'one mouth, two ears', meaning we should listen twice as often as we speak. Being a good listener can be profitable in gathering important information and feedback from clients, and that information can have significant implications on planning and organising an exercise session. Effective observation (such as being attentive to a client's body language) can provide access to important information when a client is not comfortable with expressing their feelings. The better and the more agreeable the personal trainer–client relationship is, the greater effect the personal trainer will have on the physical and mental condition of their client and the longer that they will have a professional relationship.

Even when personal trainers are apparently doing nothing, or think they are doing nothing, they are communicating. For example, when a client meets their personal trainer for the first time, they will form an opinion in the first few seconds. This first impression is based on the personal trainer's image, body language, facial expressions, voice tone and verbal content. If the client does not trust or like what they see in the personal trainer, the personal training dynamic will likely fail. For this reason the PEAP acronym provides guidelines when meeting someone for the first time (Coulson 2013):

Polite: Shake hands and state your name.

Eye contact: Maintain eye contact at all times.

Appearance: Be professional in your appearance and set an example.

Person's name: Listen carefully and remember the client's name.

The personal trainer's image, body language and facial expressions are considered *nonverbal communication*. The influence of nonverbal communication is often underestimated. Are we smiling the right amount? Is our body language in line with the message we want to convey? How is our posture? Are we walking properly? Is our attire in line with the example we want to set or the message we want to convey? The importance of these questions reinforces the need for the personal trainer to learn communication skills that are not only related to verbal communication.

Different Personal Training Environments

Prior to the last decade, personal training in Europe grew as primarily a gym or health club service. In the last decade, however, large growth has occurred in a wide variety of environments beyond the context of the gym or health club (table 3.7). Outdoor exercise sessions and those held at the worksite are growing markets for personal trainers. All environments have advantages and disadvantages, as well as intervention specifics for personal training preparation and intervention and for delivering personal training sessions (table 3.8).

Fitness Environment

The fitness environment has long been mainstream for personal training. It includes various specific settings, some of which are presented in table 3.7. Personal training in fitness settings is often an additional service for members who already pay a membership fee. For the personal trainer a fitness setting is valuable because they have access to a large volume of potential clients, more space and a large range of equipment (although this requires the personal trainer to have a wider knowledge base).

Personal training studios have also developed over recent years; this environment targets people interested in the privacy of a one-to-one situation and people who want more affordable personal training sessions that are conducted with small groups (2 to 5 clients). The disadvantage, though, is that studios are often not as well equipped as large gyms and health clubs.

In general, fitness settings have the advantage of being safe and offering emergency care and mandatory first aid in crisis situations.

Table 3.7   Personal Training Environments and Settings

Environment	Setting
Fitness	Gyms Health clubs Wellness centres Personal training studios Pilates studios
Outdoor	Urban contexts Nature contexts
Worksite	Office (small indoor facilities) Warehouses (spacious indoor facilities) Other
Home	Home equipped gym Living room or alike
Other	Hospitals Medical clinics Senior housing Spa Thermal facilities

Table 3.8   Characteristics of Personal Training Session Environments

Environments	Advantages	Disadvantages	Intervention specifics
Fitness	Safe environment directed for exercise practice Plentiful availability of exercise materials (e.g., dumbbells, kettlebells, free weights, mats, ergometers, strength training machines) Easy to apply most training methodologies and to work every muscle in the body	Closed environment that may get boring with time Usually demands an extra fee to permit access to the facilities and equipment	This is the most proficient environment for intervention. The challenge here is the large amount of different exercises and methodologies that this environment allows, which demands from the personal trainer a broad knowledge about different materials and the critical components and performance specificities of a wide range of exercises.
Outdoor	Open-air environment Easy access and free of charge An environment that may provide the client some autonomy and therefore induce longer-lasting lifestyle changes A good alternative to indoors to help change the routine and break a dull cycle for clients who feel bored working out in the gym all the time Most sustainable	More demanding in assuring the safety of the client due to the following: Wildlife, unexpected weather irregularities in nature settings Traffic and road crossing, street occasional works and repairs and voyeurs in urban areas Air, noise and even waste pollution in urban areas More difficult to have fitness equipment available	It is very important to plan ahead when training with a client outdoors: Choose the trail or specific place where the training session is to take place. Check the spot, preferably as close to the training session as possible, to identify safety issues and avoid surprises. Always carry a cell phone and design an emergency plan for any scenario. Adapt the training session to the specific spot where it will occur.

(continued)

Table 3.8 *(continued)*

Environments	Advantages	Disadvantages	Intervention specifics
Worksite	May be particularly easy to fit in daily routine May provide the client with some autonomy and induce longer-lasting lifestyle changes Usually protected from weather conditions and nature elements Highly sustainable	With the exception for large companies who have good fitness facilities within the worksite, training sessions in worksite environments usually occur in tight spaces that do not allow a wide range of exercises and methods; this is aggravated by the scarce availability of fitness equipment.	Use exercises that do not require a lot of space (e.g., stretching exercises; strength and resistance exercises: push-ups, squats, dead lifts; aerobic endurance exercises: burpees and other). Make a wide use of exercises that use only body weight for resistance.
Home	Particularly easy to fit in daily routine The client may feel safer being in their own space, contributing to the sense of comfort zone. Provide the client a lot of autonomy and may induce long-lasting lifestyle changes Protected from weather conditions and nature elements The client is encouraged to acquire affordable fitness equipment (dumbbells, mats, rubber bands and other).	With the exception for wealthier homes that have fitness facilities within them, the home environment is a lot like the worksite environment: small spaces and scarce fitness equipment. Some clients may feel that their space is being invaded, and they may not like to be pushed to work hard in this environment.	Use exercises that do not require a lot of space (e.g., stretching exercises; strength and resistance exercises: push-ups, squats, dead lifts and others; aerobic endurance exercises: burpees and other). Make a wide use of exercises that use only the body weight for resistance. The personal trainer may bring some light portable equipment to the personal training session at the client's homes (e.g., steps, rubber bands, Swiss ball, dumbbells). With time, the personal trainer may advise clients to acquire some affordable materials.

Outdoor Environment

The outdoor environment—often sought to escape routine from work or a regular gym or health club setting—is categorised as *urban settings* near or inside cities that are altered by human activity and construction (e.g., urban gardens and parks, walkways, and seafronts) and *nature settings* that have not been significantly influenced by human activity (e.g., forests, national parks, beaches and mountain trails). Two disadvantages of outdoor settings are the exposure to weather conditions and reduced safety level (if the setting was not built or modified to promote safe exercise). To improve or promote safety, the personal trainer should do the following:

- Avoid dangerous routes or places (e.g., crossing roads, unprotected elevated walkways, dangerous wildlife, and slippery floors).
- Check the location before going there with a client to identify and avoid dangerous routes and places and identify changes in the setting that reduce the safety level.
- Have an emergency plan adapted to the specific setting.
- Carry a cell phone for easy communication.

The advantages of an outdoor environment include the use of terrain inclines, elements from nature (e.g., rocks, trees) or street furniture (such as street benches, stairs or handrails) and specially built outdoor exercise stations.

Worksite Environment

Increasing evidence exists of the positive effect of physical activity on employee absenteeism (Cancelliere et al. 2011; Schultz and Edington 2007), cognition throughout adulthood (Ratey and Loehr 2011) and overall productivity (Barr-Anderson et al. 2011; Cloostermans et al. 2014). Therefore many businesses are subsidising memberships at a local gym or building fitness facilities in their corporate headquarters. From a business standpoint it makes sense that promoting healthy habits will reduce health care costs.

The worksite can present challenges to the personal trainer. With the exception of large companies that invest in fitness facilities in their corporate headquarters, most companies do not have an appropriate and especially dedicated fitness setting within their building. For this reason personal trainers often deliver personal training sessions in tight offices or small spaces with lack of equipment and versatility. Therefore the personal trainer needs to assess the specific setting (e.g., Are chairs available? Is there heavy stuff that could be lifted? Is there somewhere to hang a suspension training strap device? Is there an appropriate space for clients to lie down?) and then select the most suitable exercises based on the limitations of the space. An outdoor space may be a good alternative to offset the deficiencies of a worksite environment.

Home Environment

The home environment has similarities to the worksite environment. With the exception of large wealthy homes that may have fitness facilities within them, most houses do not have specially dedicated fitness facilities or equipment. Therefore the personal trainer must be prepared to be creative in order to deliver successful exercise sessions in smaller or non-traditional spaces that lack equipment.

Strategies for personal training in a home environment include selecting exercises that do not require a lot of space but match the intended type of mechanical or metabolic stimulus (e.g., resistance exercises: body weight only, exercises using household objects; aerobic endurance exercises: burpees or skipping or running in place).

The outdoor environment may be a good and affordable alternative setting for personal training when homes are unsuitable for exercise sessions. A fitness setting is also a good alternative; however this usually involves an extra fee. Moreover many people who look for personal training at home just want to stay in their comfort zone so that their self-confidence is high enough to accept being challenged and to engage in exercise. Some clients who prefer to do personal training at home may also mention a lack of time to go to a gym or a reluctance to meet other people.

Extending Frequent and Good Communication to Clients

Technology can help personal trainers in their job and with specific tasks related to health and fitness assessment and exercise prescription, and can be invaluable in extending the personal training sessions beyond the session itself. Technology allows the personal trainer to maintain regular contact with the client even when meeting only two or three times a week or when the client is away on business travels, work breaks or holidays. This allows a coaching style of client follow-up, and may increase adherence to both exercise and a general change in lifestyle. The use or purpose of technology commonly focuses on client assessment and exercise prescription, monitoring and entertaining the client during workouts, monitoring and managing the client's lifestyle and communication and interaction with the personal trainer.

Client Assessment and Exercise Prescription

Personal trainers may use devices such as a bioelectrical impedance, heart rate monitor, or heart rate variability monitor to assess a client's health-related fitness or make an exercise prescription. Software applications are available for most electronic devices (computers, tablets and smartphones) that may help in storing data related to exercise assessment and prescription and tracking a client's exercise progression. The use of such resources makes any personal trainer more efficient, and also allows them to dedicate more time to the client. In general technology can be extremely helpful for the personal trainer, raising the bar on professionalism and promoting the delivery of high-quality service.

Monitoring and Entertaining the Client During the Workout

During the workout session, the personal trainer can use technology to monitor a client's response to exercise. Heart rate monitors for tracking the workout's metabolic effect on the client are the most common. In addition pedometers, accelerometers, GPS-enabled tracking devices, altimetry and barometric gauges and body thermometers are also available. These devices allow the personal trainer to receive comprehensive information about what is happening during the workout (e.g., a pedometer or accelerometer provides information regarding the number of steps taken, and it may be used to calculate step rating; running speed and altimetry gauges may be used to calculate elevation changes, which may be useful for a more accurate calculation of energy expenditure). Clients may also use technology-based entertainment during the workout (e.g., a playlist on a smartphone or music-playing device). Some ergometers found in health clubs have built-in screens so that clients can watch TV or use the Internet. Entertainment strategies are particularly useful for longer and repetitive exercise sessions (e.g., walking, running or cycling). Listening to music during exercise has been proposed to have an ergogenic effect that can increase aerobic endurance exercise time up to 21 percent (Karageorghis and Priest 2012). This may be a good strategy to help clients overcome boredom and promote adherence.

Monitoring and Managing the Client's Lifestyle

A recent trend in technology is lifestyle monitoring and management devices. One common gadget is an armband or wristband that is capable of monitoring steps (pedometer), heart rate (heart rate monitor), body temperature (thermometer), sitting time (inactivity timer), light exposure (circadian rhythm monitor) and calculations of caloric expenditure. These devices can often link to software applications that analyse the collected data and offer encouraging feedback or healthy lifestyle advice.

Smartphones and tablets also have a wide range of applications that monitor lifestyle status and lifestyle progression. They often provide encouraging feedback, healthy advice and sometimes comparisons and competitions with a local, regional or global community of users (e.g., How do I rank among other users regarding the increase in daily number of steps?). This type of game-like feedback is highly motivating for some, and may be an important tool for a personal trainer. Personal trainers can also find software applications to monitor multisports, including walking, running and cycling, and to allow a client to engage in challenges that can help boost their motivation, such as running a 10K personal record or running a set distance in a month. Some applications even propose to replace the personal trainer, claiming to make fitness fun and help people stay motivated. These can be an easy way for clients to keep a personal trainer in their pocket. This may work for a small cluster of clients with an enormous drive of motivation and an unusually high level of autonomy (e.g., for personal trainers themselves!). For the majority of clients, though, the best and most sustainable option is to rely on a personal trainer's help in designing an individualised and optimised training programme that is adjusted to their particular needs.

In general personal trainers should view technology as a useful tool and a catalyst for offering high-quality personal training services, rather than a threat to their business.

Communication and Interaction With the Personal Trainer

Personal trainers can access all lifestyle data properly collected with monitoring devices and uploaded into a software application in real time. As mentioned some software applications allow clients to receive automatic feedback about their achievements. Even if the personal trainer is not interested in the software features regarding feedback and ranking, they may still use these software applications to monitor a client's lifestyle data and then send personalised feedback in an interactive fashion. This collaborative approach maintains a good personal trainer–client communication and extends the connection, as well as the commitment, far beyond the personal training session.

Personal trainers may give immediate feedback to the client whenever appropriate (e.g., to praise a client for reaching 10,000 steps in a day or to inspire a client who is sitting too often or for too long). These data can also be useful for introducing adjustments to the individualised exercise programme and for interpreting results obtained after any planned period of training. A personal trainer who makes good use of available technology is like having a support staff working 24 hours a day, 7 days a week!

Conclusion

Delivering a personal training session is a demanding and highly multidisciplinary endeavour that should be carried out by prepared and competent professionals. It requires a strong and broad theoretical and scientific background, a high level of awareness and perception, a capacity for skilful intervention and effective communication. Personal trainers must study hard and acquire substantial knowledge about a considerable number of fields, from physiology and biomechanics to psychological pedagogy and sales. High levels of awareness and perception comes from the personal trainer's motivation, but they should also support these with study and hone them with practice. Ultimately effective preparation, strong education, persistent training and mindful experience will determine a personal trainer's proficiency and success in delivering a personal training session.

Functional
Anatomy ⇒⇒⇒⇒⇒

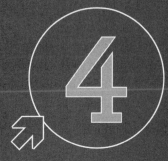

Skeletal Articulations and Joint Movement

Daniel Robbins

Mark Goss-Sampson

This chapter attempts to build on the introduction to the skeletal system that can be found in chapter 1 of *EuropeActive's Foundations for Exercise Professionals* and relates anatomy to functional kinesiology and biomechanics of the skeletal joints and movements, which occur at the joints. In order for the body to function, each of the bones must become part of a system, with each section depending on its neighbour to allow effective movement to take place. The connections between each of the bones are known as *articulations* or *joints*. The joints are held together by soft tissues, including ligaments and various connective tissues. This chapter discusses the various skeletal tissues and structures, as well as the effect of exercise, providing a foundation knowledge for exercise professionals such as personal trainers.

Connective Tissue

It is impossible to understand the role of joints in movement without a basic understanding of the connective tissues involved. Connective tissues are found all over the body and have many functions, such as connecting the epithelium (skin) to the rest of the body, storing energy reserves, transporting fluids and organic materials around the body, protecting internal organs and defending the body from infection. Considering all of these roles is outside the scope of this chapter; therefore it addresses only the role of connective tissue in relation to musculoskeletal anatomy and movement. The following are examples of connective tissue:

- *Cartilage.* This flexible connective tissue is found in many parts of the body and is more flexible than bone but less than muscle (Hamil et al. 2014). Three types of cartilage are present in the human body: elastic cartilage (found in the outer ear), hyaline cartilage (found at the end of articulating bones) and fibrocartilage (found between the spinal vertebrae and pelvis, for example). The knee, wrist, acromioclavicular, sternoclavicular and temporomandibular joints also contain a special type of fibrocartilage known as *meniscus* (Watkins 2010). The meniscus of the knee is the most well- known. Often when the joint is not stated, it is simply assumed that *meniscus* refers to the meniscus of the knee. The primary role of the meniscus is to improve joint congruity.

- *Periosteum.* This thin connective tissue layer surrounds bones. A fibrous outer layer provides protection and attachment for tendons and ligaments. The periosteum has sensory nerve endings that are particularly sensitive to tearing, the primary source of pain when bones are fractured. The periosteum also provides blood and nourishment to the cortical bone via the bone marrow (Moore and Dalley 2006).

- *Joint capsule.* This thick fibrous layer surrounds the cavities of joints, providing a sealed environment and a limit to excessive movement. The capsule produces synovial fluid, which provides lubrication within the joint as well as nutrients to joint components (Salter 1998).

- *Ligaments.* Bands of thick fibrous tissue typically connect bones to other bones and limit excessive movements. In joints these provide stability and guide joint movement. Specialised nerve receptors in both ligaments and the joint capsule respond to joint position and tension (Bear et al. 2007).

- *Tendons.* These fibrous connective tissues join muscle to bone. When muscles contract, the force they develop is transmitted through the tendon to the bone, resulting in joint movement. Specialised nerve endings known as Golgi tendon organs at the musculotendinous junction detect changes in the amount of force the tendons experience in situations such as muscle contractions and stretches (Bear et al. 2007).

All these types of connective tissue constitute the structure of joints in the skeletal system. Three types of joints are involved in human movement to a greater or lesser extent.

Joint Structure

The various joints in the body are broadly categorised into three groups:

1. Synarthrosis, or *immovable* joints formed by connective tissues between bones
2. Amphiarthrosis, or *cartilaginous* joints formed by cartilage between bones
3. Diarthrosis, or *freely movable* joints formed by soft tissues, cartilage, bones and synovial fluids (Wakefield and D'Agostino 2010)

Synarthrosis, or fibrous joints, are *immovable joints*; the bones are dovetailed together (i.e., have no joint cavity) and are bound tightly by tough fibrous tissue. Examples of these include the teeth within their sockets (known as *gomphosis joints*), as well as the sutures found between the bones making up the skull and between some long bones such as the tibia and fibula of the leg (known as a *syndesmosis joint*).

Cartilaginous joints are those where cartilage (either hyaline or fibrocartilage) forms the connection between articulating bones. These joints allow more movement than fibrous joints but less than synovial joints. Examples of these include the pubic symphysis of the pelvis, the attachment of the ribs to the ribs and the spine and the intervertebral discs. The amount of movement depends on the locations of the joint; for example, the different sections of the spine have different amount of movements in each direction (Nordin and Frankel 2012).

Synovial joints are the most common type of joint within the human body. All of the synovial joints are freely moveable and are surrounded by a synovial capsule, which produces synovial fluids to lubricate the joints. Adjacent to the joint and connective tissues are the bursae (singular form *bursa*). Bursae are sacs of fluid that act to reduce friction around the joint, for example, between tendons and bone or muscle and bone (Levangie and Norkin 2011). The areas where the different bones articulate are protected by layers of strong hyaline cartilage which is 1 to 5 millimetres thick that do not have blood supply or neural innervation (Hall 2014).

Six types of synovial joints exist that are classified by their structure and amount of movement permissible (see figure 4.1 and table
4.1):

- *Hinge joints.* With this type of joint movements are uniaxial
  (e.g., the elbow or knee), where movement occurs predominantly in one direction.

- *Pivot joints.* These involve predominantly uniaxial movements.
  One of the bones forms a perpendicular convex shape around
  the end of another bone (e.g., the top of the neck, axis and
  atlas bones), allowing the joint to rotate.

- *Saddle joints.* This type of joint allows biaxial movements. The
  surfaces are curved in a convex and concave manner (e.g., the
  thumb), allowing a wide range of movements.

- *Ellipsoidal or condyloid joints.* Biaxial movements are possible
  where an oval-shaped bone meets another with an elliptical
  cleft (e.g., the wrist and toes). This type of joint has a medium
  range of movement.

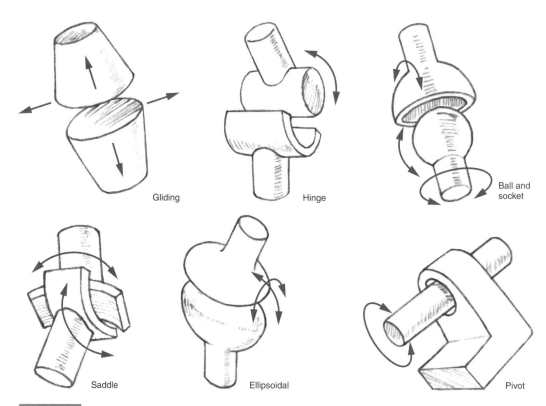

Figure 4.1 Synovial joints.

Reprinted, by permission, from P.M. McGinnis, 2013, *Biomechanics of sport exercise,* 3rd ed. (Champaign, IL: Human Kinetics),
270.

Table 4.1 Ranges of Joint Motion

Joint	Movement	Range of motion (start to end)	Variations in end ranges of motion
Shoulder	Extension–flexion	0-180°	150-180°
	Hyperextension	0-45°	40-60°
	Adduction–abduction	0-180°	150-180°
	Lateral rotation	0-90°	80-90°
	Medial rotation	0-90°	70-90°
	Horizontal abduction	30°	—
	Horizontal adduction	135°	—
Elbow	Extension–flexion	0-145°	120-160°
Forearm	Supination	0-90°	80-90°
	Pronation	0-80°	70-90°
Wrist	Extension	0-70°	65-70°
	Flexion	0-90°	75-90°
	Radial deviation	0-20°	15-25°
	Ulnar deviation	0-30°	25-40°
Thumb CMC	Abduction	0-70°	50-80°
	Flexion	0-45°	15-45°
	Extension	20°	0-20°
	Opposition	Tip of thumb to tip of #5	—
Thumb MCP	Extension–flexion	0-45°	40-90°
Thumb IP	Extension–flexion	0-90°	80-90°
#2-5 finger MCP	Flexion	0-90°	—
	Hyperextension	0-30°	30-45°
	Adduction–abduction	0-20°	—
#2-5 finger PIP	Extension–flexion	0-100°	100-120°
#2-5 finger DIP	Extension–flexion	0-90°	80-90°
Hip	Extension–flexion	0-120°	110-125°
	Hyperextension	0-15°	10-45°
	Abduction	0-45°	45-50°
	Adduction	0-20°	10-30°
	Lateral rotation	0-45°	36-60°
	Medial rotation	0-35°	33-45°
Knee	Extension–flexion	0-135°	125-145°
Ankle	Dorsiflexion	0-15°	10-30°
	Plantar flexion	0-45°	45-65°
Subtalar joint	Inversion	0-30°	30-52°
	Eversion	0-15°	15-30°
MTP	Extension–flexion	0-40°	30-45°
	Hyperextension	0-80°	50-90°
IP	Extension–flexion	0-60°	50-80°

CMC = carpometacarpal; DIP = distal interphalangeal; IP = interphalangeal; MCP = metacarpophalangeal; MTP = metatarsophalangeal; PIP = proximal interphalangeal.

Reprinted, by permission, from S. Shultz, P. Houglum, and D. Perrin, 2016, *Examination of musculoskeletal injuries,* 4th ed. (Champaign, IL: Human Kinetics), 78.

- *Gliding or plane joints.* Multiaxial movements are possible in these joints between essentially flat bones (e.g., the scapular and some of the bones in the hand). Ligaments hold the bones parallel to each other, preventing rotating movements.

- *Ball-and-socket joints.* Multiaxial movements are possible in these flexible joints where one bone forms a spherical end (socket) and the other bone a ball, allowing a wide range of multidirectional movements (e.g., the shoulder and hip).

Lever Systems

After developing knowledge of the articulations, personal trainers must learn the location at which muscles attach to the bones in order to understand the biomechanics of joint movements. When a muscle contracts the force is transmitted through its tendon to the bone, causing movement. This movement is related to lever systems (from the French word *lever*, meaning to raise). The classical definition of a lever system is one that involves a rigid bar pivoting around a fixed point (fulcrum or axis of rotation). These are used to move weight with either a pushing or, more relevantly in the skeletal system, a pulling force. Levers are defined by the relationship between the point where the force is applied, the axis of rotation and the load that is to be moved. In the musculoskeletal system, the applied force is defined as the contraction of a muscle at its point of attachment. The axis of rotation is the joint's centre and the load is the weight to be moved (i.e., limb weight or anything being held or carried, that is, *resistance*).

The perpendicular distance between the applied or load points and the axis of rotation is known as the *moment arm*. This value is relevant to the amount of muscle force required to move a load, and it is used to calculate *mechanical advantage*, or the length of the applied force arm divided by that of the load (resistance) arm. If the moment arm of the applied force is greater than the load, less force is required to move the load (mechanical advantage). If the moment arm of the applied force is less than the load, more force is required to move the load (mechanical disadvantage). In the musculoskeletal system there is a trade-off between mechanical advantage and range of motion; in particular a greater range of motion is associated with reduced mechanical advantage. Three classes of levers exist in the body: first, second and third.

First-Class Lever Systems

In this system the axis of rotation is in between the load force and the muscle force in a configuration similar to a see-saw, allowing balanced movement (see figure 4.2).

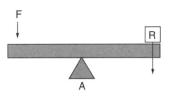

Figure 4.2 First-class lever (neck; F = fulcrum, A = muscle action, R = load).

Reprinted, by permission, from W.C. Whiting and R.F. Zernicke, 2008, *Biomechanics of musculoskeletal injury*, 2nd ed. (Champaign, IL: Human Kinetics), 77.

This configuration allows for some of the weight to be shared between that generated by the muscles and the axis of rotation. An example of this lever system is the action of the triceps brachii muscle group, which applies its contractile force to its attachment on the olecranon (a section of bone near the elbow) in extending the load of the forearm around the elbow.

Second-Class Lever Systems

In a second-class lever system the load force is in between the axis of rotation and the muscle attachment. This configuration is similar to that of a wheelbarrow, where the upward force occurs farther from the axis of rotation than the downward force from the load does, allowing small forces to lift larger weights. This system has mechanical advantage, but a reduced range of motion (see figure 4.3). An example within the body is around the ball of the foot when performing a heel

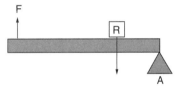

Figure 4.3 Second-class lever (ankle; F = fulcrum, A = muscle action, R = load).

Reprinted, by permission, from W.C. Whiting and R.F. Zernicke, 2008, *Biomechanics of musculoskeletal injury*, 2nd ed. (Champaign, IL: Human Kinetics), 77.

raise: The ball of the foot is the axis of rotation as the calf muscles (applied force) pull up on the heel to lift the body (load force). Another example is during a push-up: The foot is the axis of rotation whilst the muscles (applied force) are pushing against the body's weight (load force).

Third-Class Lever Systems

The body has more third-class levers than first or second. The muscle attachment is closer to the axis of rotation than to the load; therefore the applied force is closer to the axis of rotation than the load force. This configuration allows a greater range of motion and faster movements; however third-class lever joints cannot generate as much force as second-class lever joints (Chandler and Brown 2006). Examples include the action of the biceps brachii (applied force) pulling in the forearm (load force) around the elbow (axis of rotation) or the hamstrings contracting to flex the knee (see figure 4.4).

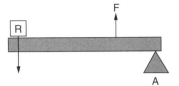

Figure 4.4 Third-class lever (elbow; F = fulcrum, A = muscle action, R = load).

Reprinted, by permission, from W.C. Whiting and R.F. Zernicke, 2008, *Biomechanics of musculoskeletal injury,* 2nd ed. (Champaign, IL: Human Kinetics), 77.

Although the lever systems are very good at explaining individual joint motions, remember that joints very rarely work in isolation. This is particularly true in movements in a straight line, such as pushing or pulling (Aaberg 2006). However, in exercise personal trainers must consider what is happening and how it can be related to other activities, such as daily living or recreational activities. One approach to this form of analysis is to compare *open* and *closed chain kinetic movements*. Open chain movements can be defined as an exercise where the distal segment, such as the hand or foot, is free to move in space without resistance. An example of an open chain exercise is the leg extension machine, or most pulley based exercise. These movements can be very muscle specific, and therefore are good for bodybuilding or rehabilitation exercises. Closed chain movements can be defined as movement where the distal segment is fixed against a resisting object, such as the floor, a wall or part of an exercise machine (for example the leg press machine). These movements are sometimes considered functional movements.

Effects of Resistance Training on Joints

Resistance training produces significant improvements, such as increases in bone density and tendon and ligament strength and stiffness, resulting in improved joint function and reduced injury potential (Whiting and Zernicke 2008). All joint components respond positively to increased mechanical stimuli and force loading as long as the forces do not exceed the individual tissue's functional limits (Farrell et al. 2011).

Normal adult bone is in a state of homeostasis that is maintained by balanced activity between osteoclasts (which break down bone) and osteoblasts (which produce new bone). Repetitive bone loading, as seen in resistance training, has been shown to increase the activity of osteoblasts, particularly at points of stress, leading to increased bone strength, density and calcium retention. The primary location of osteoblast activity is on the outside of bones, in the periosteum; the osteoclast activity occurs on the inside surface in the trabecular bone. This pattern of change allows bone to adapt to the imposed demands without losing the relative structure (i.e., diameter of the hollow centre to the total bone diameter) whilst increasing girth, stiffness and strength (Watkins 2010). Note that during activity, particularly in sport, the demands experienced by the body are often not symmetrical. For example, Nazarian and colleagues (2010) investigated the effect of regular participation in football (soccer) on the bone mineral density of the legs. Their findings indicated that the bones in players' non-dominant legs had significantly higher bone mineral densities than those of their dominant legs.

A similar response to loading is seen in the collagen fibres of the connective tissues, particularly the major structural components of ligaments and tendons involved in force transmission. Repeated resistance training causes tissue adaptation by increasing the diameter of individual collagen fibrils, the number and density of the fibrils and tissue stiffness (force transmission capacity per unit of tissue stretch). All of these changes lead to the increase in size, strength and stiffness of ligaments and tendons.

Conclusion

Human movement typically occurs from a co-ordinated effort from groups of joints. To understand the movements each joint is capable of, readers must first understand joint anatomy. The structure and interaction between hard and soft tissues (e.g., bone, cartilage, tendon and ligaments) dictates how much movement can occur and the directions in which the movement occurs. Effective and safe exercise relies on movements being completed within the individual range of motion available at each joint. Knowledge of the structure of joints also provides an insight into whether a joint is more suited to producing force or faster contractions. Synovial joints are capable of more movement than other joint types, though synovial joints are also less stable than cartilaginous or immovable joints. Out of all the synovial joints third-class lever systems allow greater range of motion and faster movements, although they cannot generate as much force as joints defined as second-class lever systems. Consistent movement, such as exercise, results in structural changes in both the soft and hard tissues creating joints, leading to increased size, density and strength.

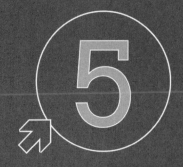

Injury Prevention

Pauline Jacobs

John van Heel

Musculoskeletal injuries are one of the most common problems people of all ages face on a daily basis. From muscle pulls to back problems, the typical lifestyle of inactivity and bad posture predisposes us to a whole range of problems. This chapter shows some of the most important diseases and injuries and provides practical information and recommendations for personal trainers.

Osteoporosis

Beginning at around age 35 in both men and women, calcium is lost, causing bones to become less dense. Osteopenia is a condition in which bone mineral density (BMD) is lower than normal, and it is considered a precursor to *osteoporosis*, which is a disease of bones in which BMD is reduced, bone microstructure is disrupted and the actual proteins in bone are altered.

Besides age, inactivity also leads to these changes in the skeletal system (National Institutes of Health 2000; Lewis and Bottomly 2007). During later years, these changes in bone mass can result in osteoporosis.

Changes in the Skeletal System

Osteoporosis is defined as a skeletal disorder, characterised by compromised bone strength predisposing a person to an increased risk of fracture. Osteoporosis can lead to a reduction of weight-bearing capacity and increased possibility of spontaneous fracture. The incidence of fracture, especially in the lumbar vertebrae, hips (neck of femur) and wrists, is high in people with osteoporosis, and it increases with age and inactivity (National Institutes of Health 2000; Lewis and Bottomly 2007).

Bone strength primarily reflects the integration of bone density and bone quality (see figure 5.1).

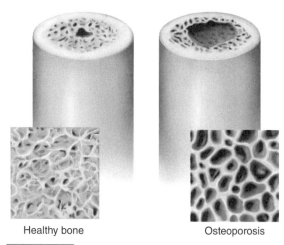

Healthy bone   Osteoporosis

Figure 5.1 Bone density depending on age.

- *Bone density* is determined by peak bone mass and amount of bone loss and is described in terms of bone mineral density (BMD).

- *Bone quality* refers to architecture, turnover, damage accumulation (e.g., microfractures) and mineralisation (National Institutes of Health 2000; Lewis and Bottomly 2007).

Effects of Exercise on Bone Health

Regular physical activity has specific effects on bone health. Strong evidence suggests that physical activity early in life can maintain or increase BMD (National Institutes of Health 2000; Lewis and Bottomly 2007), and therefore can prevent people from developing osteoporosis.

In older age exercise has a modest effect on slowing the decline in BMD (Body et al. 2011; Friedlander et al. 1995; de Kam et al. 2009; Księżopolska-Orłowska 2010; Magkos et al. 2007; National Institutes of Health 2000; Snow-Harter et al. 1992). Exercise late in life, even beyond age of 90 years, can increase muscle mass and strength. This results in an improved function and delayed loss of independence, and thus contributes to quality of life (National Institutes of Health 2000; Lewis and Bottomly 2007).

People who participate in resistance training have a higher bone mineral density than those who do not (Layne and Nelson 1999). Some evidence suggests that high-impact exercises combined with resistance exercises increase BMD more than aerobic exercise does (Body et al. 2011; Friedlander et al. 1995; de Kam et al. 2009; Księżopolska-Orłowska 2010; Magkos et al. 2007; Snow-Harter et al. 1992). Resistance exercise is also recommended for improving muscle strength and balance. Other recommendations involve combining resistance exercise and weight-bearing aerobic exercise such as walking and jogging (Body et al. 2011; Friedlander et al. 1995; de Kam et al. 2009; Księżopolska-Orłowska 2010; Magkos et al. 2007; Snow-Harter et al. 1992).

The primary goal of exercise is to reach optimal peak bone mass (de Kam et al. 2009). The secondary goal is to improve muscle strength, co-ordination and balance, which in turn decrease the frequency of falls (de Kam et al. 2009). To reach these goals clients should combine aerobic exercise and strength training for the big muscle groups (prime movers) in the body (Body et al. 2011; Friedlander et al. 1995; de Kam et al. 2009; Księżopolska-Orłowska 2010; Magkos et al. 2007; Snow-Harter et al. 1992). For people who undergo a decline in BMD, adequate intake of calcium and vitamin D is recommended (National Institutes of Health 2000; Lewis and Bottomly 2007). Finally it is very important to practise exercise safety to prevent falling and possible fractures.

Musculoskeletal Injuries

Musculoskeletal injury refers to damage of muscular or skeletal systems, usually due to a strenuous activity (Hootman et al. 2002). Research suggests that musculoskeletal pain is more common now than it was 40 years ago (Harkness et al. 2005). In one study, roughly 25 percent of approximately 6,300 adults received a musculoskeletal injury of some sort within 12 months, and 83 percent of those injuries were activity related (Hootman et al. 2002).

Proper posture ensures that the muscles of the body are optimally aligned at the proper length–tension relationships necessary for efficient functioning of force couples. Proper posture helps the body produce high levels of functional strength. Without it the body may degenerate or experience poor posture, altered movement patterns and muscle imbalances. These dysfunctions can lead to common injuries such as ankle sprains, tendinitis and lower back pain.

Spinal Injury Prevention

The spinal column is one of the most important body parts. Without it you could not support yourself upright or perform many complex functions. A healthy spine optimises your body's transmission of energy and allows you to go through your daily tasks with ease and comfort.

Spinal Curvature

A normal spine is shaped like the letter S (see figure 5.2). In a normal spine four types of spinal curvatures are important in terms of balance, flexibility, and stress absorption and distribution. Spinal curves are either kyphotic or lordotic. A kyphotic curve is anteriorly concave and convex posteriorly. A lordotic curve has curves in the opposite direction. Clients should maintain the correct degree of curvature during postures and movements. See figure 5.2 for normal curvatures.

The curves of the spine are important because they actually allow the spine to support more weight than if it were straight. This is because the curves increase resistance for axial compression. Any excessive exaggeration of the spine's curves results in compression of the discs and compensation in the kinetic chain, for example, through muscle synergies. This places stress and strain on the entire back.

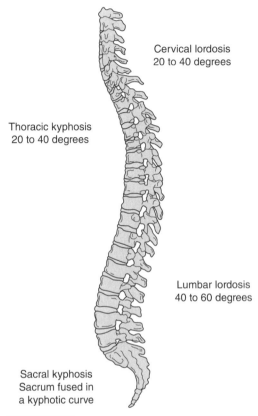

Cervical lordosis
20 to 40 degrees

Thoracic kyphosis
20 to 40 degrees

Lumbar lordosis
40 to 60 degrees

Sacral kyphosis
Sacrum fused in
a kyphotic curve

Figure 5.2 Spinal curves and their normal degree of curvature.

Intervertebral Discs and Shock Absorption

Between the vertebrae, the spinal column contains 23 cartilaginous pads called *intervertebral discs*. These discs are located between each of the 33 vertebrae. Their main function is to act as shock absorbers and provide separation between and stability among the vertebrae. The intervertebral discs are also responsible for the flexibility of the spine. The only way to strengthen the discs is to stimulate the spine. This can be done by movement, which increases blood circulation and the fluid content of the discs (Buckwalter 1995). An intervertebral disc has a soft, jelly-like centre called the *nucleus pulposus* and a tough outer casing called the *annulus fibrosis*. During non-weight-bearing activities (like sleeping) the discs expand as they soak up fluid, increasing the length of the spine overnight. However the pull of gravity during the day results in compression fatigue that causes the average adult to lose height as the day goes on. Sometimes the outer annulus can tear, allowing the inner jelly to leak out. If the leak presses on the spinal cord or on a nerve, it can cause pain to radiate into the leg or arm (see figure 5.3).

Measurements of disc pressure over the last 20 years in more than 100 individuals have demonstrated how the load on the lumbar disc varies with the position of the subject's body and during the performance of various tasks. Table 5.1 shows the approximate load on the L3 disc in a person weighing 70 kilograms (Nachemson 1981). During activities like sit-ups, forward bending and holding

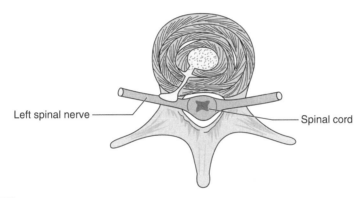

Left spinal nerve ———— ———— Spinal cord

Figure 5.3   A leak from the nucleus pulposus of an intervertebral disc can place pressure on the spinal cord.

Table 5.1   Approximate Load on the L3 Disc in a Person Weighing 70 Kilograms (Nachemson 1981)

Position	Force
Standing at ease	500 N
Lying on your back	250 N
Sitting with lumbar support	400 N
Sitting, no back support	700 N
Coughing	600 N
Sit-ups	1,200 N
Forward bend 20°	600 N
Forward bend, 40°	1,000 N
Forward bend, 20° with 20 kg	1,200 N
Forward bend, 20° rotated 20°, 10 kg	2,100 N
Holding 5 kg, arms extended	1,900 N

weight with extended arms, the forces on the back increase to a huge extent. This is why personal trainers must instruct their clients to hold the weight close to the body during lifting and to perform lifts with flexed knees.

Personal trainers should advise clients to always use correct technique when sitting and lifting in their daily lives to prevent injuries. They should also instruct clients to always lift weights holding the weight close to the body and keeping the knees bent and the back straight. During sport these forces can even be stronger, so personal trainers must always pay attention to their client's posture when performing an exercise.

Muscle Synergies of Spine Posture

Important components of the spine are the supporting muscles (i.e., adjoining muscles) and ligaments. Muscles are used for the following three basic functions:

1. Creating and maintaining the curves of the spine
2. Resisting the force of gravity and straightening by contracting and exerting compressive force on the spine
3. Supporting the spine

Several recent studies have shown that core training decreases the risk of spine injuries (Sahrmann 1993; O'Sullivan et al. 1997; Hodges and Richardson 1998). People who have chronic lower back pain activate their core muscles less and have a lower endurance for stabilisation. The core musculature helps protect the spine from harmful forces that occur during functional activities.

Weak muscles can result in poor posture, and faulty movement can induce pathology (Sahrmann 1993). To help clients avoid injuries personal trainers should always include core training in their training programmes. Personal trainers should also make sure the client's muscle synergy is in balance (i.e., their ROM is at the appropriate length) and train all the muscles involved in the synergy. To relieve unnecessary stress and compression on the discs, clients should improve their posture and strengthen their core muscles.

Abnormal Degrees of Curvature

Three types of abnormal curvature of the spine exist: excessive lordosis, kyphosis and scoliosis. All three of these can be either congenital or developed after birth in any stage of life. The following section discusses what these types of curvature involve and how personal trainers should operate when training clients with abnormal curvatures.

Lordosis is an exaggerated lumbar curve in the spine, also known as a swayback. A lordosis often develops later in life due to muscle weakness or bad posture. Some muscles around the hip and spine become tight and some become weak and stretched, causing an imbalance. This is due to the position of the tight and weak muscles (see figure 5.4).

An excessive kyphotic curve is also often developed later in life. Exercise techniques are similar for both an excessive kyphotic curve in the thoracic spine and lumbar lordosis. Typically with a kyphotic curvature in the upper back, an exaggerated lordosis also appears in the cervical spinal column. The upper back appears curved with rounded shoulders; the scapulae are protracted and elevated and the chin pokes forwards rather than being tucked in (see figure 5.5).

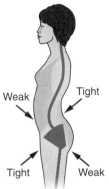
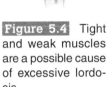

Figure 5.4 Tight and weak muscles are a possible cause of excessive lordosis.

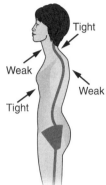

Figure 5.5 Tight and weak muscles are a possible cause of excessive kyphosis.

Muscle Imbalance

Muscles in the movement system of the core have a tendency to become tight, and those in the stabilising system of the core can become weak. If the movement system is strong and the stabilisation system is weak, the kinetic chain senses an imbalance, and forces are not transferred or used properly. This leads to compensation, synergistic dominance and inefficient movements. Static and dynamic stabilisation of the lumbo-pelvic-hip complex can prevent an excessive lordosis (Hodges and Richardson 1997).

In the early 1970s Janda identified three basic compensatory patterns:

- Lower crossed syndrome (LCS): a postural distortion syndrome characterised by an anterior tilt to the pelvis (arched lower back)
- Upper crossed syndrome (UCS): a postural distortion syndrome characterised by a forward head and rounded shoulders
- Layer syndrome: essentially a combination of UCS and LCS that is characterised by alternating patterns of tightness and weakness, indicating long-standing muscle imbalance pathology

Lower Crossed Syndrome

In lower crossed syndrome (figure 5.6), tightness of the thoracolumbar extensors on the dorsal side crosses with tightness of the iliopsoas and rectus femoris. Weakness of the deep abdominal muscles ventrally crosses with weakness of the gluteus maximus and medius.

Specific postural changes seen in LCS include anterior pelvic tilt, increased lumbar lordosis, lateral lumbar shift, lateral leg rotation and knee hyperextension. If the lordosis is deep and short, then imbalance occurs predominantly in the pelvic muscles; if the lordosis is shallow and extends into the thoracic area, then imbalance occurs predominantly in the trunk muscles.

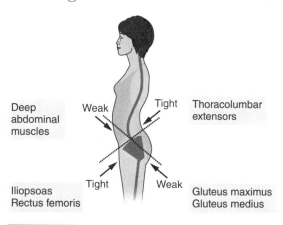

Figure 5.6 Tight and weak muscles in lower crossed syndrome.

The purpose of training in this case would be to strengthen the stabilising system of the core. The core-stabilisation system needs sustained contractions (6 to 20 seconds) in order to improve intramuscular co-ordination and motor-unit recruitment within a muscle. Performing a lunge, squat or overhead press with excessive spinal lordosis is an example of compensation that results from weak core stabilisation.

Upper Crossed Syndrome

In upper crossed syndrome (figure 5.7), tightness of the upper trapezius and levator scapula on the dorsal side crosses with tightness of the pectoralis major and minor. Weakness of the deep cervical flexors ventrally crosses with weakness of the middle and lower trapezius. Specific postural changes are seen in UCS, including forward head posture, increased

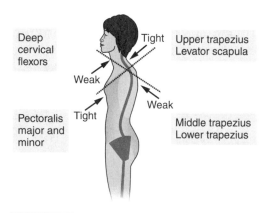

Figure 5.7 Tight and weak muscles in upper crossed syndrome.

cervical lordosis and thoracic kyphosis, elevated and protracted shoulders, and rotation or abduction and winging of the scapulae (Page et al. 2010). In this case the stabilising system of muscles is also needed for improving intramuscular co-ordination and motor-unit recruitment.

Scoliosis

Scoliosis is often congenital, and the severity varies a lot between people. Most of the time training approaches for clients with scoliosis are based on preventing additional injuries. Scoliosis is a three-dimensional condition involving spinal changes in different planes, and it can consist of one curve in the coronal plane (*C* shape) or two curves in the coronal plane (*S* shape) and a possible torsional curve (see figure 5.8). Physical exercises, if correctly administered, can prevent a worsening of the curve (Fusco et al. 2011).

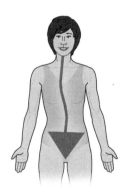

Figure 5.8 Scoliosis is a three-dimensional abnormal curvature of the spine.

The aims of exercise for clients with scoliosis are as follows:

- Correction of the scoliotic posture
- Improved mobility of the whole spine
- Increased length of the musculature of the whole body
- Strengthened core muscles (upper back and lower back; Fusco et al. 2011).

For correction of the scoliotic curves, asymmetric exercises are recommended. Clients should try to achieve equal strength on both sides (Fusco et al. 2011).

Shoulder Stabilisation

Anterior shoulder dislocation is a common injury in an athletic population, particularly among young men competing in contact sports. Anterior dislocation accounts for up to 96 percent of all shoulder dislocations (Goss 1988). The shoulder joint usually refers to the glenohumeral joint. This ball-and-socket joint allows the arm to rotate in a circular fashion or to hinge out and up, away from the body. The ball is the rounded surface of the humerus and the socket is formed by the glenoid fossa, the dish-shaped portion of the lateral scapula. The shallowness of the socket and relatively loose connections between the shoulder and the rest of the arm allow the arm to have tremendous mobility. The disadvantage of this mobility is that the shoulder is much easier to dislocate than most other joints in the body.

To preserve the stability of the shoulder joint and thus prevent it from being displaced, both good passive and active stability are crucial. Passive stability involves the ligaments and the capsule of the glenohumeral joint (see figure 5.9). The capsule and ligaments cannot be trained, and people with bad passive stability (e.g., due to hypermobility) must improve their active stability by training the kinetic chain of muscles around the shoulder joint.

Active Stabilisation of the Shoulder

The stabilisation of the scapula has a crucial role in proper shoulder function during movements (Kibler 1989). An imbalance among scapular stabilising muscles, rotator cuff muscles and the prime movers of the shoulder joint causes active glenohumeral instability.

Muscles concerned with stabilisation and rotation of the scapula include the trapezius, rhomboid, levator scapulae and the serratus anterior. Muscles that provide glenohumeral joint stabilisation include the intrinsic muscles of the rotator cuff: the subscapularis, supraspinatus, infraspinatus and teres minor. The prime movers of the shoulder joint include the extrinsic muscles of the shoulder joint: the deltoid, biceps and triceps muscles.

The purposes of training for people with high risk of shoulder displacement due to instability are as follows (listed in order of priority):

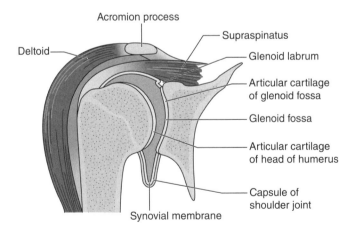

Figure 5.9   The glenohumeral joint. Note the shallowness of the scapular part of the ball-and-socket joint. Ligaments and the articular capsule stabilise the joint passively.

- Stabilisation training of the scapular stabilising muscles
- Stabilisation training of the rotator cuff muscles
- Strength training of the prime movers of the shoulder joint (Kibler 1989; Voight and Thomson 2000)

Training of shoulder stabilisation should start at the base of the kinetic chain. This usually means correcting any strength or flexibility deficits that exist at the cervical and thoracic level (Kibler 1989; Voight and Thomson 2000).

The most organic way to reorganise and re-establish normal firing patterns for the scapula is with the exercises that involve closed chain activities (Kibler 1989). They reproduce the normal physiological patterns of cocontractions of the scapular stabilising muscles and of the muscles of the rotator cuff (Kibler 1989; Prokopy et al. 2008).

Open chain activities may be initiated on the base established by the isometric and closed chain activities (Kibler 1989).

Ligamentous Damage

Several ligaments are present in every joint in the human skeleton. Ligaments are considered the primary restraints of the bones constituting the joint. As joints go through their range of motion, with or without external load, the ligaments ensure that the bones associated with the joint travel in their prescribed anatomical tracks, maintain full and even contact pressure of the articular surfaces, prevent separation of the bones from each other by increasing their tension, as may be necessary, and ensuring stable motion (Solomonow 2009).

In order to fulfil this function, ligaments must possess immense mechanical tensile strength. Ligaments are defined as dense connective tissue, and they are made up of a protein substance called collagen.

Ligament sprains can be classified according to their severity (Guo and De Vita 2009):

- *Grade 1.* The ligament is overstretched. A few collagen fibres are damaged, producing a local inflammatory response. This is characterised by pain over the affected ligament.
- *Grade 2.* A more extensive number of collagen fibres are damaged, producing a more marked inflammatory response. This moderately affects the joint stability.
- *Grade 3.* A complete rupture of the ligament occurs and causes severe joint instability. Surgery may be necessary to restore joint stability.

Risk of Tears and Sprains

The organisation of collagen fibres gives the ligament its tensile strength. Ligaments consist of closely packed, parallel collagen fibres. Various degrees of undulation (or helical shapes) appear to form along the axis of each fibre at a resting length. Short cross fibrils also connect the axial fibres to each other. As axial stretching of a ligament is applied, fibres or bundles with a small helical wave appearance straighten first and begin to offer resistance (increased stiffness) to stretching. As the ligament is further elongated, fibres or fibre bundles of progressively larger helical wave straighten and contribute to the overall stiffness. Overall this recruitment process gives rise to a non-linear length–tension relationship of a ligament (see figure 5.10; Solomonow 2009). Damage is defined as a reduction in straight collagen fibre's stiffness, which occurs at randomly defined stretching points of the collagen (Guo and De Vita 2009).

Fast stretching of ligaments, such as in high-frequency repetitive motion or in sport activities, can result in high incidents of ligamentous damage or rupture (Guo and De Vita 2009). Research has mainly studied the incidence of ankle sprains and sprains of the ligaments of the knee because of their high incidence in sport. The conservative treatment during a sprain includes RICE treatment (rest, ice, compression, elevation; Fong et al. 2009) and balance and strengthening exercises (Verhagen et al. 2004).

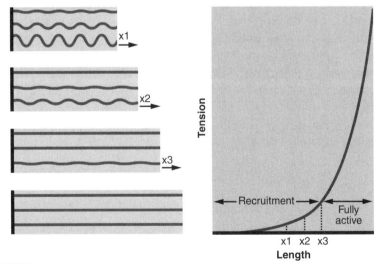

Figure 5.10 The length–tension behaviour of a ligament is shown on the right. On the left, the progressive recruitment of collagen fibres is shown for several elongations (Solomonow 2009).

Reprinted from *Journal of Body Work and Movement Therapies,* Vol. 13(2), M. Solomonow, "Ligaments: A source of musculoskeletal disorders," pgs. 36–154, copyright 2009, with permission from Elsevier.

Excessive Non-Functional Movement During Activities

Excessive non-functional movement (e.g., exaggerated rotation of the torso and internal rotation of the hip or knee during running) places exaggerated stress on the kinetic chain and increases the risk for sprains in knees and ankles. Personal trainers must always prevent their clients from performing non-functional movement.

Assessment is vital for analysing the client's movements. Personal trainers should pay attention to their clients' way of performing the instructed exercise. They should correct any non-functional movements or implement exercises that can improve the client's technique. An exercise programme should always start with exercises that fit the client's physical capacity at that point. For example, it is better to let clients run at a speed that they can perform in with correct technique, that is, without any compensations. In case of an injury, personal trainers should immediately apply the RICE treatment.

Conclusion

Personal trainers must focus on preventing injuries. This chapter discusses the contributions of physical activity to good health for the elderly, particularly its positive influence on osteopenia and osteoporosis. Good posture also helps prevent injuries, both during training and in daily life.

Other injuries can be prevented or improved by paying attention to muscle imbalances during physical training in the lower back and the shoulder girdle, keeping the lower extremity in good condition and preventing excessive non-functional movement (ligamentous injuries).

6

Muscular System

Anders Nedergaard

This chapter provides information about the different types of muscular contraction and their effects on training adaptations, as well as the way muscles can be influenced by different training modalities. In addition it emphasises the relevance of the hip flexor muscle iliopsoas and the thoracolumbar fascia, which are very important in core stability training. The chapter should be read in conjunction with chapter 2 of the book *EuropeActive's Foundations for Exercise Professionals.*

Contraction Types and Their Characteristics

Muscle action and exercises can be classified based on their mechanical and bioenergetic properties. These contraction types can be assigned to individual muscles as well as to the different parts of exercises. In general the contraction type assigned to a part of an exercise corresponds to the contraction type in the primary muscles of an exercise, i.e., during the concentric phase of a bench press, the pectoralis muscle also works concentrically. Some of the contraction types occur in everyday physiological movement, whereas others can only occur in certain forms of specialised equipment, described as artificial contraction (Knuttgen and Kraemer 1987) in the following section on contraction classifications.

Physiological Types

This section describes the classifications of normal contractions that occur in everyday movement.

Concentric

Concentric work occurs when muscle contraction results in a shortening of the muscle. Myosin ATPases crawl down the actin molecule, reducing the length of the muscle. Concentric work is the contraction modality in which the muscle has the greatest capacity for sustained energy output. On the other hand, concentric work has the lowest capacity for force production. The faster the muscle is contracting, the lower its capacity for force production, a phenomenon illustrated by the curve describing the force–velocity relationship (see figure 6.1; Bottinelli et al. 1996; Bottinelli et al. 1991; Gordon et al. 1966; Miller et al. 2005; Thorstensson et al. 1976).

Certain forms of exercise require almost exclusively concentric work, such as bicycling and swimming. This is even true for certain momentum-based resistance exercises such as power cleans or snatches, where the eccentric phase is either omitted (e.g., by dropping the bar) or executed passively (i.e., with absent or minimal intended activation).

During concentric exercise (but not eccentric exercise) muscle fibres and motor units are recruited in accordance with Henneman's size principle, which dictates the recruitment hierarchy of motor units. The size principle specifically states that motor units are recruited in order of increasing size and speed profiles with increased demands (Henneman et al. 1965; McPhedran et al. 1965a; 1965b). This is not the case for eccentric exercise, which is explained more in a following section. The majority of energy required during a full repetition of any movement is spent during the concentric phase, because energy expenditure is much bigger at this point than during the isometric or eccentric phases. Therefore the majority of the metabolic stress produced during exercise occurs during the concentric phase.

Isometric

Isometric work occurs when the muscle contracts without changing length. This occurs most of the time in stabilising, tonic musculature like the trunk muscles (when standing), during the stabilisation done by synergists when other muscles are performing dynamic movement and in the transition between the eccentric and concentric phases (or vice versa). Force production potential in isometric activity is higher than in concentric contractions, which is evident in the force–velocity curve, but is lower than in eccentric contractions (see figure 6.1). Because isometric contractions are by definition almost always sustained, they are subjected to mechanical stress–induced occlusion (described in further detail in the corresponding section). This means that during isometric exercise fatigue sets in earlier than during movements without sustained loading, thereby changing activation patterns. During fatigue motor units shut down and take microbreaks, necessitating the activation of higher threshold motor units. Therefore, even at low loads, sufficient fatigue calls for activation of motor units otherwise restricted to very high loads.

Eccentric

Eccentric work occurs when the muscle lengthens during activation (i.e., the muscle yields to external mechanical forces). When yielding under force, work is produced by gravity or existing momentum; as a consequence eccentric work costs very little energy (LaStayo et al. 2000; Lindstedt et al. 2001; Ryschon et al. 1997). The force–velocity curve shows that during eccentric contraction higher forces can be produced than during concentric or isometric contractions (see figure 6.1; by definition eccentric work corresponds to negative contraction speeds). In eccentric work force potential increases with decreasing contraction speed (i.e., increasing negative contraction speed).

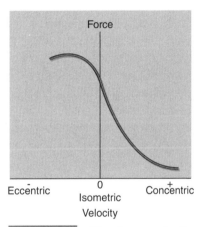

Figure 6.1 The force–velocity relationship.

Reprinted, by permission, from W.C. Whiting and S. Rugg, 2006, *Dynatomy: dynamic human anatomy* (Champaign, IL: Human Kinetics), 77.

The activation strategies used by the nervous system during eccentric exercise are different from those specified by the size principle (Enoka 1996). Although it is still not well understood, part of this different recruitment strategy is selective activation of high-threshold motor units (i.e., those normally only recruited under very high loads).

Eccentric exercise stimulates muscle damage and remodeling much more than the other contraction modalities. During exercise with combined contraction types, the majority of the stimulus towards muscle damage is produced in the eccentric part of the movement. When compared to concentric-only exercise, eccentric-only exercise results in more hypertrophy, but not as much as a combination of concentric and eccentric exercise. This is why activity with very pronounced eccentric components tends to result in more muscle damage and soreness than activities with less pronounced eccentric components do. Good examples of eccentric-dominant activities are running, walking or running downhill and most resistance training.

Artificial Types

These contraction classifications occur reproducibly only under lab conditions, when working against mechanical devices capable of operating at fixed forces or velocities. They are explained here because they are frequently used in physiological testing and in scientific literature. Note that they are not mutually exclusive with physiological contractions (i.e., an isokinetic exercise still contains concentric and eccentric phases).

Isokinetic

Isokinetic work occurs when a contraction occurs at a constant velocity throughout the movement. Thus isokinetic work can also be concentric or eccentric, and isometric work is by definition isokinetic. When the velocity of the movement is fixed, the variable component in the isokinetic work produced is the force of contraction; the external object will move with the same speed, no matter how much force is applied to it. From a pragmatic perspective, isokinetic devises are used to test the amount of force that can be produced at different speeds.

Isotonic

Isotonic work is done when a contraction occurs at a constant force throughout the movement. Hence isotonic work can also be concentric, isometric or eccentric. Resistance-exercise movements that are executed at constant speed and in straight lines (e.g., leg press) would be termed *isotonic.*

Acute Muscle Adaptations to Different Training Types

Performing a particular type of exercise produces a range of stimuli at the myocellular level. In response to those stimuli, muscle adapts acutely in a number of ways to become more effective at producing that type of exercise. This is accomplished as the cells of the muscle build the structures necessary for producing that kind of exercise and for resisting the kind of fatigue it induces.

Exercise Hyperaemia

All types of muscle exercise lead to muscle hyperaemia, or an increased flow of blood through the muscle. When exercise begins or activity levels otherwise increase, blood flow to the muscles increases immediately (within 5 seconds) by as much as tenfold through a localised vasodilatory response. This is limited to the muscle being worked. Obviously this increases delivery of oxygen and nutrients as well as clearance of metabolites, thereby improving performance of the muscles in question. The mechanisms behind this effect are poorly understood, but the effect is thought to be mediated by reductions in blood oxygen saturation, decreases in pH (hormonal or locally) or systemic neurotransmitters (Clark et al. 2008; Joyner 2006; Poole et al. 2008; Sheriff 2005).

The phenomenon known as *the pump* in fitness circles describes a temporary pooling of blood in the exercising muscle that occurs particularly during unaccustomed, fatiguing resistance exercise and disappears less than an hour after exercise. Although this phenomenon may appear to be related to exercise hyperaemia, most researchers agree that it is not. The pump phenomenon is very poorly described from a scientific point of view, and has been described only very superficially. Researchers do not know where in muscle this swelling is situated (i.e., if it is intracellular or extracellular or in the vessels themselves). Scientific inquiry has also not explored whether the accumulation of water in the muscle is a passive phenomenon, like osmosis, or an active one, such as from active pumping of water.

So far no scientific findings imply that the pump is necessary for adaptation, and it may not even be indicative of a particularly positive training response. The importance commonly ascribed to this phenomenon in fitness circles is possibly explained by its consistent appearance during anabolic steroid use.

Mechanical Stress–Induced Occlusion

During sustained isometric work or resistance training with continuous muscle tension, blood flow is compromised because the intramuscular pressure is higher than the intravessel pressure in the venules and capillaries of the muscle. This occlusion starts at loads corresponding to approximately 20 percent of (mechanical) intensity and increases with increasing intensity. Compromised blood flow limits the delivery of oxygen and nutrients and the removal of electrolytes and metabolites. Ultimately energy production becomes compromised during occlusion due to deprivation of oxygen and accumulation of metabolites. This changes the bioenergetics of muscle work towards (lactic) anaerobic, even though the energy produced in the muscle would normally be aerobic.

This means that continuous loading, such as during intentionally slow repetitions of resistance exercises, leads to increased fatigue relative to the amount of work produced or the amount of load used. Because fatigue accumulation and fatigue-associated metabolites and electrolytes also contribute to the adaptive response to exercise, sustained loading techniques may provide an adequate stimulus for hypertrophy in the absence of optimal external loads, such as during bodyweight training.

Muscle Damage and Delayed-Onset Muscle Soreness (DOMS)

Whenever any combination of strenuous, unaccustomed and eccentric exercise is performed, a degree of muscle damage may develop. This is a condition that progresses over the course of 2 to 10 days, but most commonly lasts only 2 to 4 days. It is associated with the hallmarks of inflammation: soreness, heating, swelling and reddening (although that may be hard to see). During muscle damage the molecular structures of the muscle cells are disrupted, meaning that cellular contents spill out into the blood. Visual inspection may reveal periodic striations of skeletal muscle.

Changes in Protein Degradation and Synthesis

Following exercise the muscle starts to build structures responsible for making it bigger, stronger, more fatigue resistant and capable of faster metabolism, such as muscle myosin, mitochondrial biogenesis and creatine kinase or calcium stores. This process can be measured as increases in protein synthesis following exercise. Exercising also causes damage to intracellular structures in the muscle, requiring some cleaning up and necessitating protein breakdown. Thus, following exercise both protein breakdown and synthesis increase, with synthesis increasing more than breakdown, resulting in an increase in net protein synthesis. Elevations in synthesis and breakdown usually peak 24 to 48 hours after exercise and return to baseline within 72 hours, although muscle soreness may persist for longer. By far the majority of adaptations take place within the first two days following the stimulus.

Diminishing Returns, Repeated Bout Effect

With repeated exercise bouts, the degree of muscle damage and the DOMS experienced becomes smaller. This means that the muscle has begun protecting itself from damage. This phenomenon is called the *repeated bout effect*. In parallel, the adaptive response to each training bout becomes smaller (Phillips et al. 1999). This protection against training is the reason why periodisation and progressive overload are necessary to produce continued adaptations.

Chronic Muscle Adaptation to Training

Sustained exercise results in an accumulation of musculoskeletal adaptations that increase performance in a manner specific to the inducing stimulus. This ranges from hypertrophy to changes in substrate stores and expression of metabolic enzymes.

Strength

Almost all types of training produce some strength increase in the untrained individual. This strength increase is specific to the position of flexion or extension, range of motion, contraction speed and degree of fatigue in which training is performed, but with significant carryover to neighbouring degrees of said factors. This increase is governed in part by changes in neuromuscular efficiency and in part by structural changes of the muscle, particularly hypertrophy.

Changes in strength can also manifest in structural adaptations outside of hypertrophy. Changes in sarcomere and fascicle length can contribute to optimisation of force–length relationships at discrete muscle lengths without necessarily involving hypertrophy, whilst improved motor drive and stretch reflex reactivity contribute to neuromuscular function (Aagaard et al. 2001; Kraemer et al. 2002).

Hypertrophy

Training of sufficient mechanical intensity, range of motion and muscle fatigue eventually results in hypertrophy (or increase in size) of muscle fibres. In principle gross muscle hypertrophy can be caused by hyperplasia as well as hypertrophy. In humans all available evidence strongly suggests that a contribution from hyperplasia is insignificant and therefore that fibre hypertrophy is the overwhelmingly dominant factor (Bolster et al. 2004; Schoenfeld 2010).

Thus, when the muscle grows, it does so by increasing the amount of contractile protein and the size and number of myofibrils inside the muscle fibres. Since these components fill 95 percent of the muscle fibres they are the only relevant contributor to increases in muscle size. The total contribution to muscle volume from variable components such as glycogen or intramuscular fat stores is less than 15 percent of total volume in normal muscle, making them dispensable in the context of gross muscle hypertrophy.

The amount of connective tissue in the muscle increases in proportion to the muscle cells, so the ratio of muscle fibre to connective tissue is maintained with hypertrophy. As discussed previously the eccentric part of a movement contributes more to hypertrophy than the concentric part does, but a combined stimulus has been shown to work better.

The fast Type II muscle fibres respond with hypertrophy more easily than the slow Type I fibres do. With 3 months of resistance training, 25 percent hypertrophy can commonly be seen, and in extremely trained individuals hypertrophy in excess of 100 percent can be observed.

Metabolic Adaptations

With exercise the metabolic profile of the muscle changes to accommodate the bioenergetic demands of exercise. These adaptations are specific in providing the metabolic apparatus to supply energy for short bursts of activity, intermediate-length bursts or sustained energy production. They can manifest as changes in levels of metabolic enzymes, levels of membrane electrolyte transport enzymes, capillarisation and storage of glycogen or intramuscular fat.

Exercise of extremely short duration (e.g., 100-metre sprints) depends solely on glycolysis and creatine phosphate pools. Therefore performing 100-metre sprinting as exercise results specifically in upregulation of glycolytic enzymes and creatine kinase. Triathlon, on the other hand, depends mostly on metabolism of fat and therefore produces more pronounced adaptations in the form of upregulation of enzymes related to beta oxidation and the Krebs cycle.

Endurance exercise modalities tend to manifest adaptations that favour long-term muscular endurance and oxidative metabolism like increased capillarisation and increased glycogen and intramuscular fat storage, whereas short-term, higher intensity exercise modalities tend to manifest in more hypertrophy, improved glucose and creatine metabolism, higher glycogen stores and improved expression of sodium–potassium channels, reducing potassium efflux during muscular fatigue (see table 6.1; Gibala and McGee 2008; Holloszy and Coyle 1984).

Table 6.1   Adaptations to Exercise

		Energy system adaptation	Fatigue resistance adaptation	Structural changes
Very short-term energy production (alactic anaerobic)	1-10 s	↑Creatine kinase ↑Creatine pools	–	↑Hypertrophy
Short-term energy production (lactic anaerobic)	10-60 s	↑Glycolysis (hypertrophy)	↑Tolerance to changes in pH	↑Hypertrophy
Intermediate-term energy production (anaerobic-aerobic)	1-5 min	↑Glycolysis ↑TCA cycle	↑Glycogen storage ↑Tolerance to changes in pH	↑Capillarisation
Long-term energy production (aerobic)	5-60 min	↑TCA cycle	↑Glycogen storage	↑Capillarisation
Very long-term energy production (aerobic)	60+ min	↑Beta oxidation ↑TCA cycle	↑Fat oxidation (sparing of muscle glycogen)	↑Capillarisation

Muscle Functions of the Hip and Thoracolumbar Fascia

The muscles of the hips and lower part of the torso constitute what is commonly referred to as the *core*. The biomechanical function of the core is important for health and optimal performance in sport. In terms of sport most athletic activities depend on force transfer from the lower body to the upper body, or vice versa, such as throwing, sprinting, wrestling and kicking. Inefficient force transfer severely impairs overall movement performance.

In health the importance of the core's function is most prominently shown when it is inadequate, which manifests as back pain. Thus personal trainers must recognise the core as an important area for training, either for restoring optimal functionality and relieving back pain or for maintaining good posture and mobility. The muscles in the hips and lower torso are not very popular in personal training programmes, possibly because they do not contribute to any sort of aesthetic improvement like, for example, the abdominal muscles.

Iliopsoas

The iliopsoas consists of two muscles, the iliacus and the psoas major. The psoas major originates on the L1 through T12 vertebrae, whereas the iliacus originates on the iliac fossa of the pelvis. Both of them converge towards the insertion on the lesser trochanter of the femur (see figure 6.2). Thus the iliopsoas produces hip flexion and external rotation of the hip.

Due to the excessive chair sitting common in the Western world, the iliopsoas frequently becomes tight, creating excessive pull on the pelvis and lumbar vertebrae and contributing to excessive extension of the lumbar spine (lordosis), which may contribute to back pain.

Although hip flexion and flexion of the spine are functionally related (in the anterior muscle sling) in human movement, imbalances between the hip flexors and spine flexors (the abdominal muscles) are common. Specifically this is because tightness increases

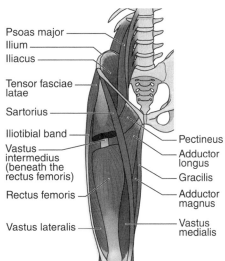

Figure 6.2 The iliopsoas muscle group consists of the iliacus and the psoas major.

pull on the spine. If this imbalance is left unchecked by the flexing pull of the abdominals, it causes excessive stress on the lower back during exercises in which hip or spine flexion occurs. In these cases personal trainers should focus on reducing the pull of the iliopsoas by stretching it and by performing exercises where spinal flexion without movement of the hip is emphasised.

Thoracolumbar Fascia

The thoracolumbar fascia (TLF) is a fascia structure covering the lower back. It envelops the erector spinae and the quadratus lumborum totally, and it is divided into three layers (see figures 6.3 and 6.4). The posterior and middle layers surround the erector spinae, whilst the anterior and middle layers surround the quadratus lumborum. Along the lateral edges the transversus abdominis and obliques insert along the superolateral aspect and the latissimus dorsi inserts along the inferolateral aspect. Thus the TLF transmits forces from all these muscles. Its most important function is to stabilise the spine in transmitting extensor forces from the erectors, but it also transmits forces that produce spinal rotation and lateral flexion and rotational forces from the hips and lower body to the upper body (the posterior oblique muscle sling) as well as to the posterolateral muscle sling. The posterior oblique muscle sling transmits forces between the gluteal muscles and the latissimus dorsi on the contralateral side.

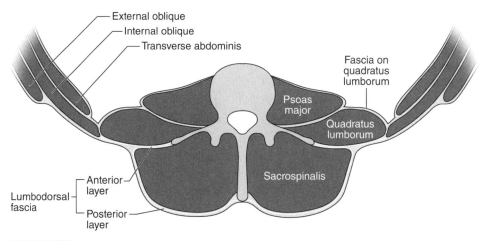

Figure 6.3 Transverse section showing the structure of the thoracolumbar fascia, covering the erector spinae (at this vertebral level, the sacrospinalis) and the quadratus lumborum.

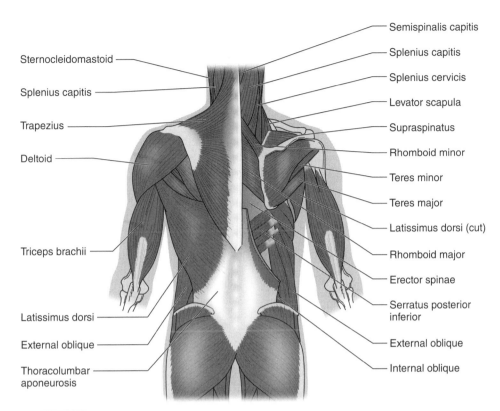

Sternocleidomastoid

Splenius capitis

Trapezius

Deltoid

Triceps brachii

Latissimus dorsi

External oblique

Thoracolumbar
aponeurosis

Semispinalis capitis

Splenius capitis

Splenius cervicis

Levator scapula

Supraspinatus

Rhomboid minor

Teres minor

Teres major

Latissimus dorsi (cut)

Rhomboid major

Erector spinae

Serratus posterior
inferior

External oblique

Internal oblique

Figure 6.4 Anatomical location of the thoracolumbar fascia in the posterior aspect.

Conclusion

In summary the skeletal muscle organ is a complex hierarchical system that can produce work efficiently, both intensely for short periods of time and at lower intensity for sustained periods. This dual ability is manifested at both the macroscopic structural level and all the way down to the cellular level. Furthermore the muscle tissue displays a remarkable ability to rapidly change performance in response to exercise across a wide range of modalities.

In personal training the core muscles, especially the iliopsoas and the thoracolumbar fascia, are very often neglected, although they play a key role in improving performance and restoring good positioning in this area.

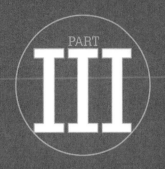

PART

III

Physiology →→→→→→

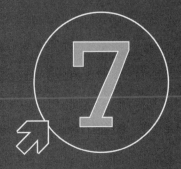

Energy Systems

Francesco Bertiato

Simonetta Senni

Why is oxygen so important in the production of energy? To answer this question you need to understand how cells, especially muscle cells, produce energy. Energy is the ability to perform work, and work is the transfer of energy from one system to another. When a muscle contracts it generates a force. The energy used to produce this contraction comes from a special substance inside the cell called ATP (adenosine triphosphate). In the production of muscular work, ATP is the fuel; the more quickly and efficiently the muscle cells can produce ATP, the less fatigued the muscle becomes. Although there are stores of ATP and another compound called phosphocreatine (PCr) within the muscle, these reserves are limited. When the stores are depleted, the muscle must be able to resynthesise ATP to continue to produce work.

The high-energy compounds ATP and PCr are a form of chemical energy extracted from sugar, fat and protein and subsequently used to produce mechanical work during muscle contractions. Muscle cells can replenish ATP by using three different biochemical pathways and a series of chemical reactions.

Three Energy Systems

The body has three energy systems. The first system is the *anaerobic alactic energy system*. It is the simplest system, and it is important because it relies on the high-energy ATP and phosphocreatine contained in the cells. This system does not require oxygen (anaerobic) and does not form lactic acid (alactic). It produces a high output but for a very short time; thus it has an extremely limited capacity.

During the first few seconds of high-intensity activity, for example a sprint, ATP levels are maintained and PCr declines rapidly due to being used in the rebuilding of the ATP supply. When the sprinter reaches a state of exhaustion, ATP and PCr stores are very low, and thus can no longer provide the energy for more contractions. Therefore the body's ability to maintain ATP levels from PCr is limited. When running at maximal intensity, stores of ATP and PCr can supply the energy needs of muscles for a short time, about 3 to 15 seconds. Recovery is usually at 50 percent after 1 minute, and full recovery should occur after 2 minutes. After that the muscles need to rely on a different process, such as the glycolytic and oxidative combustion of fuels, to produce another form of energy.

The second system is the *anaerobic lactic acid energy system*, where, in the absence of oxygen, glucose breaks down into lactic acid. Here ATP is produced when special glycolytic enzymes break down blood glucose or stored glycogen. This is termed the *glycolytic system*. *Glucose* refers to the sugar circulating in the bloodstream. Blood glucose is made when the digestive system breaks down carbohydrates. The glycogen synthesised from glucose (glycogenesis) is stored in the liver or muscle until it is needed. This system does not produce large amounts of ATP. Despite this limitation the combined action of the ATP/PCr and glycolytic systems permit the muscles to generate force in the event of a limited oxygen supply. These two systems are used during the first few minutes of high-intensity exercise. The major limitation of anaerobic glycolysis is that it leads to an accumulation of lactic acid in the muscles.

The anaerobic systems can ensure an energy supply for activities that do not exceed a maximum duration of 2 minutes. Any additional demand for energy by the body must be supplied by the aerobic system.

The third system of cellular energy is the *aerobic energy system*. This is the most complex of the three energy systems. The process by which the body converts energy using oxygen to break down fuel is called *cellular respiration*; it is an aerobic process due to the use of oxygen. This oxidative production of ATP takes place inside special types of cells called mitochondria. During long-term exercise the muscles require a constant supply of energy to continue performing.

Unlike the other two energy systems, the aerobic system has the ability to produce energy for a prolonged period.

The aerobic metabolism is therefore the process mainly involved in resistance activities where oxygen must be transported to the muscles in order to carry out the activity.

The three energy systems do not work independently. When a person exercises at maximum intensity, whether a short sprint (less than 10 seconds) or a long-distance run (more than 30 minutes), all three systems contribute to their energy needs. The combined systems help to produce fuel on a continuous basis over the duration of the activity. This permits different ways of supplying energy to the person performing.

Acute Variables and Energy Systems

Although an energy system can be predominant in response to a specific muscle activity (e.g., the system alactacid for the maximal repetition or the aerobic one for the marathon), all three energy sources can provide the ATP request from the body at any time. Therefore the system of phosphates also intervenes when the body is at rest, whilst aerobic sources are also involved during the lift ceiling. In fact, even in a resting state, muscles produce a small amount of lactate that is then released into the blood. During a marathon, even if most of the energy is made by the aerobic system by oxidative sources, a small part of the energy required originates from the anaerobic systems of phosphates and lactate.

Although all three systems provide energy to obtain a part of the ATP required for any activity, changing some parameters commonly called *acute variables* (e.g., the duration or the intensity of the exercise) will of course change the predominance of one of the three systems. Acute variables are usually identified as specific components in order to define how each exercise should be performed regarding a specific training objective.

They represent the measure of fatigue inducted to the body. From this point of view, it is easy to understand that acute variables form the foundation of a personal training programme.

To help personal trainers correctly prescribe strength training exercises and understand adjustments that occur in energy systems and muscle fibre types, table 7.1 provides a full overview of the interactions of acute variables depending on the following four goals:

- Muscular endurance
- Hypertrophy
- Maximal strength
- Power

Table 7.1   Correlation of Each Acute Variable on Different Types of Goals

Acute variables of training	Definition	Muscular endurance and stabilisation	Hypertrophy	Maximal strength	Power adaptations
Repetitions	One complete movement of a single exercise	12-20 reps at 50–70% 1RM	6-12 reps at 75–85% 1RM	1-5 reps at 85–100% 1RM	1-10 reps at 30–45% 1RM
Sets	A group of consecutive repetitions	1-3 sets of 12-20 reps at 50–70% 1RM	3-5 sets of 6-12 reps at 75–85% 1RM	4-6 sets of 1-5 reps at 85–100% 1RM	3-6 sets of 1-10 reps at 30–45% 1RM
Training intensity	A client's level of effort compared to their maximal effort, which is usually expressed as a percentage	50–70% 1RM	75–85% 1RM	85–100% 1RM	30–45% 1RM
Repetition tempo	The speed at which each repetition is performed	Slow repetition tempo: One example would be 4 s eccentric, 2 s isometric, 1 s concentric (4/2/1).	Moderate tempo: One example would be 2 s eccentric, 0 s isometric, and 2 s concentric (2/0/2).	Fast or explosive tempo	Fast or explosive tempo that can be safely controlled
Rest interval	Time used to recuperate between sets	0-90 s rest	0-60 s	3-5 min rest	3-5 min rest

Adapted from Aaberg 2007 and Clark, Lucett, and Sutton 2011.

From the cardiorespiratory training point of view, note that the acute variables can have specific adaptations, primarily on energy systems but also on the skeletal muscles and the nervous system. Table 7.2 classifies the training zones related to acute variables that determine these variations. Furthermore, for an effective prescription, the table equations help personal trainers estimate the optimal heart rate in a specific area.

Table 7.2 Correlation of Cardiovascular Intensity, Acute Variables (Time and Intensity) and Calculation of Heart Rate Zone

Intensity	Energy system	Acute variables (time > intensity)	Equation
III. 86–95% HRmax	Anaerobic alactic	III > 30 s II > 2 min I > 1 min	Upper limit: [(HRmax – HRrest) × .95] + HRrest – lower limit: [(HRmax – HRrest) × .86] + HRrest
II. 76–85% HRmax	Anaerobic lactic acid	II > 1 min I > 30 s	Upper limit: [(HRmax – HRrest) × .85] + HRrest – lower limit: [(HRmax – HRrest) × .76] + HRrest
I. 65–75% HRmax	Aerobic	II > 1 min I > 30 s	Upper limit: [(HRmax – HRrest) × .75] + HRrest – lower limit: [(HRmax – HRrest) × .66] + HRrest

HRmax (maximum heart rate) is determined by the method of subtracting the client's age from 220, unless a direct measure is available.

Adapted from Clark, Lucett, and Sutton 2011 and Katch, McArdle, and Katch 2010).

Personal trainers should understand that each client's goals require different ingredients when designing an appropriate training plan. The aforementioned conditions for acute variables are a framework for understanding the needs of each client and optimising their favourite training methodologies in order to help them reach their goals within a personal training programme.

Effects of EPOC and Interval Training on Metabolism

The body's ability to estimate the oxygen demand of the muscles is not perfect. During the initial part of exercise, the oxygen transport system (breathing and circulation) is not immediately able to satisfy the oxygen demand of the involved muscles. It takes several minutes before oxygen consumption reaches the required level (steady state) and the aerobic process becomes fully functional. Because the demand for oxygen and oxygen availability are different during the transition from rest to activity, an oxygen deficit is created, even during low-intensity exercise. The oxygen deficit is calculated by taking the difference between the oxygen required for a given work intensity (steady state) and the oxygen consumed at that time. Despite the lack of oxygen, the muscles fail to produce the necessary ATP through anaerobic pathways. On the contrary, during the initial minutes of recovery, the demand for oxygen does not decrease immediately even if the muscles are no longer working hard; thus oxygen consumption remains temporarily high. This excess volume of oxygen, one that exceeds the normal consumption at rest, was traditionally called *oxygen debt*. Today another term is commonly used for this excess of oxygen consumption after exercise: excess post-exercise oxygen consumption (EPOC). EPOC is the surplus of oxygen from what is usually consumed at rest. Just think of what happens after a physical effort such as running to catch a departing bus or running up a few stairs: Heart rate raises and you breathe heavily. After several minutes of recovery, pulse and breathing return to normal.

For many years the EPOC curve was described as having two distinct components: a fast initial component and a slower secondary component. According to the classical theory, the fast component of the curve represented the oxygen needed to replenish the used ATP and PCr stores. During oxygen deficiency, the high-energy phosphate bonds of the ATP–PCr compounds are broken to provide the energy required. During recovery it is necessary to restore these bonds through the oxidative process in order to replenish energy stores.

It was thought that the slow component of the EPOC curve represented the removal of lactate accumulated in the tissues, or the process of replenishing muscle glycogen. On the basis of this theory, both the fast and the slow components of the curve were considered an expression of anaerobic capacity during exercise. It was believed that analysing oxygen consumption after exercise would enable the amount of anaerobic activity performed to be estimated. However, more recent studies indicate that the classical interpretation of EPOC is too simplistic. For example during the initial exercise period, some oxygen is borrowed from the oxygen stores (haemoglobin and myoglobin). This oxygen must then be returned in some way during recovery. Therefore, EPOC depends on many factors, not just on the reconstruction of ATP and PCr and the elimination of lactate produced by the anaerobic metabolism. EPOC physiological mechanisms have thus yet to be clearly defined.

Interval training is a training method that includes peaks of high-intensity exercise followed by rest periods. It is also known as *Fartlek* (Swedish for speed play). Interval training involves pushing your body beyond its aerobic threshold for a certain amount of time then returning to aerobic conditioning with the aim of improving performance (speed, strength and aerobic endurance). The aerobic threshold is the point at which the body shifts from burning a higher percentage of fat and a higher percentage of carbohydrate, generally around 85 percent of maximum heart rate. Thus, unlike a normal aerobic routine where you maintain the same pace or intensity, interval training uses segments of high-intensity activity to allow you to work for a shorter period of time with recovery. It is much easier to maintain than an entire workout at a high intensity. Another advantage is that this method of training can be used for all types of exercises. Not least, aerobic training intervals offer a safe and comfortable way to exit your comfort zone and make your training more challenging and effective (see figure 7.1). It is also been shown to improve the health of patients with chronic obstructive pulmonary disease and metabolic syndrome. The main benefits of an interval training workout are as follows:

- *Increased aerobic endurance.* Interval training actually trains your heart to pump more blood to the muscles and to utilise oxygen more efficiently.
- *More efficient workouts.* Interval training workouts are great time-savers, allowing you to perform a complete session in a shorter period of time.
- *Greater fuel efficiency.* Interval training improves the body's use of fat and carbohydrate.
- *More power and muscular endurance.* Working at high intensities raises your lactate threshold and can improve your performance.
- *Weight loss.* Studies show that interval training, even at a moderate intensity, may burn greater amounts of fat and, if the intensity is sufficient, can increase fat burning post workout.

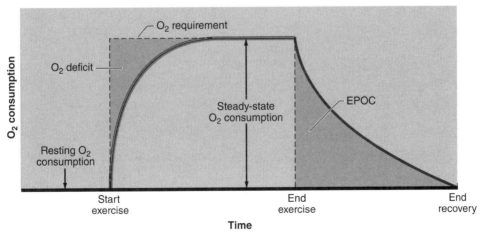

Figure 7.1 O_2 consumption.

Reprinted, by permission, from W.L. Kenney, J.H. Wilmore, and D.L. Costill, 2015, *Physiology of sport and exercise,* 6th ed. (Champaign, IL: Human Kinetics), 129.

Fat Burning

As stated earlier aerobic activity seems to be one of the most recognised pathways for fat burning. Moreover the aim of burning fat in the fastest way possible is a common goal for many who exercise. It is well known that regular exercise and aerobic endurance training are considered to be the best types of physical activity for weight loss. Despite the large number of studies attempting to determine the optimal methods for this goal, the exact protocol for ensuring general body weight maintenance has not yet been found. Carbohydrate and fat are the two main sources of fuel used in sustaining energy requirements during exercise. Their specific use, and percentage of each substance required, depends on exercise intensity. The carbohydrate is oxidised in specific high-intensity activities, whilst increased fat consumption occurs in an operating range between low- and moderate-intensity exercise.

Within the past few years the term *FatMax* has gained popularity. This refers to the peak point on the fat oxidation curve, and it is dependent on exercise intensity. Jeukendrup and Achten (2001) evaluated a range of maximum fat utilisation (see figure 7.2) defined as around 63 percent of $\dot{V}O_2$max in trained individuals and around 50 percent of $\dot{V}O_2$max in sedentary individuals.

Familiarity with the characteristics of fat burning is very important. In addition to traditional evaluations for an exercise goal that can

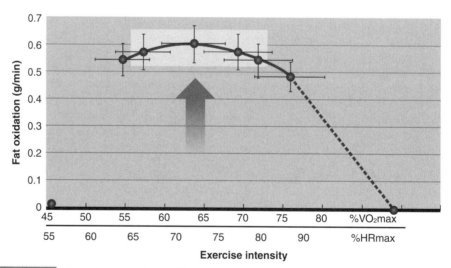

Figure 7.2 Exercise intensity and fat oxidation.

Reprinted, by permission, from J. Achten, M. Gleeson, and A.E. Jeukendrup, 2002, "Determination of the exercise intensity that elicits maximal fat oxidation," *Medicine & Science in Sports & Exercise* 34(1): 92-97.

provide an aesthetic improvement of the physical shape, this concept can be applied for clients who have problems with metabolism management due to pathological problems. From this perspective, obese clients or those suffering from diseases such as diabetes can benefit from the management of training loads that significantly enhance exercise efficiency.

METs and Calories

The metabolic cost of different physical activities is another way to determine the right exercise intensity. The appropriate range of intensity is usually between 60 and 80 percent of the client's maximum functional capacity. Since we now know the energy cost of most physical activities, those that fall within the prescribed range may be a useful way of improving cardiorespiratory function. A MET, or metabolic equivalent, is a unit for expressing the energy cost of different physical activities. It is a multiple of energy consumption at rest, and the value of one MET is equivalent to the resting metabolic rate. A MET is equivalent to an oxygen consumption of 3.5 millilitres per kilogram of body weight per minute:

$$1 \text{ MET} = 3.5 \text{ ml} / (\text{kg} \times \text{min})$$

Moreover, it has been conventionally accepted that the value of 1 MET corresponds directly to 1 kilocalorie per kilogram of body weight per hour:

$$1 \text{ MET} = 1 \text{ kcal/kg/h}$$

By using these formulas, it is possible not only to indirectly determine a client's exercise intensity, but also to evaluate the energy expenditure on the basis of exercise duration and body mass. Ainsworth and colleagues (2011) developed a fundamental approach for assessing the intensity of exercise and activity. Table 7.3 shows some of these items, divided by intensity in METs and their numerical values.

For example, a person weighing 70 kilograms who performs an exercise classified as 10 METs for 15 minutes, has a corresponding O_2 consumption of 35 millilitres / (kilograms of body weight $\times$ minutes). The caloric consumption is then calculated as follows:

$$10 \text{ METs} = \text{kcal/kg/h}$$
$$\text{Kcal} = 10 \times 70 \times (15/60)$$
$$= 175 \text{ kcal}$$

Table 7.3   MET Value per Type of Physical Activity

Physical activity	MET
Light-intensity activities	<3
Sleeping	.9
Watching television	1.0
Writing, desk work, typing	1.8
Walking at 2.7 km/h (1.7 mph): strolling very slowly on level ground	2.3
Walking, 4 km/h (2.5 mph)	2.9
Moderate-intensity activities	3-6
Bicycling, stationary, 50 watts, very light effort	3.0
Walking 4.8 km/h (3.0 mph)	3.3
Calisthenics, home exercise, light or moderate effort, general	3.5
Walking 5.5 km/h (3.4 mph)	3.6
Bicycling <16 km/h (10 mph), leisure, to work or for pleasure	4.0
Bicycling, stationary, 100 watts, light effort	5.5
Vigorous-intensity activities	>6
Jogging, general	7.0
Calisthenics (e.g., push-ups, sit-ups, pull-ups, jumping jacks), heavy, vigorous effort	8.0
Running, in place	8.0
Rope jumping	10.0

From Ainsworth et al. 2011.

Note that the published MET values (as in the previous example) are derived from experimental studies, and thus are indicative averages. Moreover the level of intensity at which a client performs a certain type of exercise (e.g., walking pace, running speed) will diverge from the standard reported MET values obtained from experimental conditions. More importantly the actual energy expenditure will differ according to the client's overall level of fitness.

Methods for Monitoring Exercise

Exercise intensity is perhaps the most critical factor in ensuring the success of a programme aimed at improving aerobic conditioning. The intensity of an activity can be defined as the energy level required for the performance. Intensity can be achieved through specific mechanisms provided by energy producers and deliverers. The term *work intensity* cannot be understood in a general sense, but it must always have a relative meaning, and will differ among clients. In absolute terms, some exercise intensities (e.g., 150 beats per minute) can be very difficult for one client but less demanding for another. The amount of work to be performed should be determined from the evaluation of specific tests and the client's health and fitness history. Generally the calculation of a given activity intensity needs to be based on heart rate or oxygen consumption (expressed as a percentage of the client's maximum functional capacity) or on data derived from or directly related to these values.

The limit of maximal heart rate (HRmax) depends on the client's health status or other individual characteristics, as well as the method of calculation or estimation. Personal trainers can choose from several methods of calculating the ideal heart rate for a workout (i.e., the frequency that must be achieved and maintained during the training session, which allows the best benefits without health risks).

Fox method: A load is set that allows exercise to be performed at a certain percentage of maximal heart rate (HRmax), which is conventionally calculated by subtracting the age of the client from 220:

$$HRmax = 220 - age$$
$$HR\ workout = \%\ HRmax$$

This method is widely known for its convenience, and it is internationally recognised as a quick and easy way of calculating maximal heart rate. However, note that some inaccuracies exist for people who tend to have an extremely high (tachycardia) or low (bradycardia) heart rate (HR). In both these cases using the formula 220 – age to estimate the value of HRmax could be inaccurate. Using the formula in the first case would generate an underestimated value and in the second an overestimated one, resulting in an inappropriate workload by default or excess (Fox 3rd et al. 1971).

Karvonen method: Here, it is first necessary to calculate what is called heart rate reserve (HRR), which is defined as the difference between the maximal heart rate (HRmax) and resting heart rate (HRrest). The heart rate for the workout will be the sum of a certain percentage of the HRR and the HRrest:

$$HRR = HRmax - HRrest$$
$$HR\ workout = HRrest + \%HRR\ at\ rest$$

A common criticism of the Karvonen method is the variability of heart rate at rest, whose values change greatly depending on the time of day it is measured, posture, emotional stress and environmental conditions. To increase the accuracy of the method, HR should be recorded at rest for several days and at several times of day under standardised conditions.

Gellish method: From a scientific point of view, this method has been proclaimed as an innovation in maximal heart rate calculation. It is closely related to the Fox method, and thus is also criticised for inaccuracy. It is based on the following calculation:

$$\text{HRmax} = 207 - (.7 \times \text{age})$$
$$\text{HR workout} = \% \text{ HRmax}$$

As with the Fox method, the maximal heart rate determines the percentage of the workload. The Gellish method is more precise than the Fox method.

It is not important which method of calculation the personal trainer uses because the HR workout is just one of many physiological responses monitored during training.

In terms of efficacy and safety, namely to determine whether a client responds in an appropriate way to the prescribed exercise, personal trainers must understand how to use the rating of perceived exertion (RPE) scale, another tool for internal and subjective evaluation of physical intensity. This type of subjective evaluation consists of a numerical scale that corresponds to certain levels of fatigue and stress, ranging from a minimum value, identified as an extremely light workout, to a maximum value corresponding to an extremely heavy workout. This scale was designed and introduced by Borg in the early '60s, and ranges from 6 (no exertion at all) up to 20 (maximal exertion; Borg 1970). It is an important method for monitoring heart rate during exercise.

Personal trainers should ask their clients how they would assess their personal feeling of exertion. The use of the Borg scale is particularly important for people for whom monitoring heart rate is problematic and unreliable, for example for those who are taking drugs such as beta-blockers that inhibit an increase in heart rate. When dealing with non-specific training goals, exercise intensity should always be between 13 (mild) and 14 (hard enough), reaching 15 (heavy) in a more advanced phase of training. Individual subjectivity is a remarkable disadvantage of this method.

A linear relationship exists between RPE and HR, and both are directly related to work intensity. Hence the RPE scale provides useful information on the extent of subjective stress during exercise. Adding a zero to each number on the RPE scale roughly relates to the heart rate for a given level of physical work. For example a score of 6 or 7 at rest reflects a frequency of 60 or 70 beats per minute; a score of 19 or 20, a frequency of 190 or 200 beats per minute. Table 7.4

Table 7.4 Relationship Between % HRmax, % HRR and Rate of Perceived Exertion Evaluations

HRmax	HRR	RPE	Intensity classification
<35%	<30%	<10	Very light
35–59%	30–49%	10-11	Light
60–79%	50–74%	12-13	Somewhat hard
80–89%	75–84%	14-16	Hard
>90%	>85%	>16	Very hard

Adapted from McArdle, Katch, and Katch 2005.

illustrates the relationship between some of the previously discussed methods, and therefore provides a scheme for classifying intensity.

Due to the linear relationship with HR, RPE increases with workload and fatigue and decreases in proportion to heart rate. Once a personal trainer has assessed the client's training adaptation, the RPE level allows the personal trainer to understand how the client responds and when it is time to increase the intensity. Clients quickly learn to regulate their physical effort based on the subjective feeling of fatigue. The Borg scale is very useful in helping clients determine the correct intensity of exercise, especially when no other control mechanisms are available, or if the client has a special constitution.

The talk test is another method of measuring the correct exercise intensity if a heart rate monitor is not available. It primarily assesses the client's ability to talk during the workout. People who are able to converse whilst working out are applying an appropriate intensity (ACSM 1998). If clients can speak comfortably, they are probably somewhere around the low to middle range of their HR workout (or the level 14-15 on the Borg scale).

Experts generally suggest that people should not be breathless during their workouts. However, when performing interval training or a short, high-intensity workout, being somewhat breathless is necessary. Obviously if a client feels dizzy or lightheaded, they should slow down or stop exercising.

Use of Energy From Nutrients

The energy required to meet the demands of the body at different percentages of intensity derives from the oxidation of carbohydrate (muscle glycogen and plasma glucose), protein and lipids (fatty acids in adipose tissue and muscle triglycerides).The main factors that determine which of these three energy substrates are used by muscles during exercise are type of exercise (continuous or intermittent), duration and intensity.

When performing low-intensity physical activity (between 25 and 30 percent of $\dot{V}O_2$ max), the required energy mainly comes from lipid metabolism by releasing fatty acids from adipose tissue triglycerides and intramuscular triglycerides. In this case glycogen is not a crucial contribution to energy production. Fatty acids are transported via the bloodstream, bound to a protein called albumin and then released into the muscles in order to form the substrate for oxidation. The maximum activation of fatty acid metabolism is reached after 20 to 30 minutes of exercise. The mobilisation of fatty acids from adipose tissue into the bloodstream to the cells and then into the mitochondria is a rather slow process.

In physical activity of mild or moderate intensity (50 to 60 percent $\dot{V}O_2$max), the role of plasma fatty acids declines. Energy derived from the oxidation of muscle triglycerides is then increased so that both sources are contributing equally to energy expenditure. Thus the contribution of fatty acids in absolute terms remains constant. For exercise of up to 20 minutes, 40 to 50 percent of the energy is supplied by muscle glycogen, whereas the rest comes from lipids and small amounts of protein. If the exercise lasts for longer, the liver is no longer able to sufficiently release glucose into the bloodstream to be delivered to the muscles, and blood sugar levels fall (45 mg/dl during 90 minutes of strenuous exercise). Fatigue occurs when there is an extreme depletion of glycogen in the liver and muscles irrespective of the availability of oxygen.

For high-intensity physical activity (75 to 90 percent of $\dot{V}O_2$max), the intensity cannot be continued for more than 30 minutes, even for well-trained people. Catecholamines and glucagon are released, and the insulin secretion is inhibited. During this type of activity, up to 30 percent of the energy demand is covered by the plasma glucose, whereas the remaining 70 percent mostly comes from muscle glycogen (1 hour of activity leads to the depletion of stores by 55 percent). The high energy demand also causes an increase in production of lactic acid, which accumulates in the muscles and blood and inhibits the lipolysis in adipose tissue.

Conclusion

A limiting factor in sport performance is the availability of oxygen. In low oxygen conditions, glucose and the phosphate reserves in the muscle are the only sources of usable energy. Anaerobic glycolysis yields 20 times less oxygen than aerobic glycolysis does, and causes the production of lactic acid, which is a metabolite responsible for muscle fatigue. For a given workload, the higher the $\dot{V}O_2max$, the higher the contribution of fat as an energy source. A workout that improves $\dot{V}O_2max$ therefore also increases the body's ability to use fat as a primary energy source.

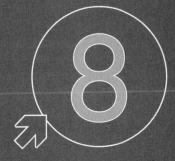

Cardiorespiratory System

Christoffer Andersen

A functional cardiorespiratory system is vital to human health and quality of life. This system is quick to adapt to acute increases in oxygen demands to support ATP resynthesis with a rapid increase in both pulmonary ventilation and cardiac output. On one hand long-term training can further increase the cardiorespiratory system's ability to handle these demands. On the other hand physical inactivity and chronic stress can lead to serious health issues within the cardiovascular system. The content of this chapter is of vital importance because personal trainers need learning outcomes about the cardiovascular and cardiorespiratory systems stated in their related educational standards. Regarding the cardiovascular system the chapter deals with the functional anatomy of the heart, the cardiac cycle and the function of the blood vessels. It also presents information on coronary heart diseases as well as the effects of physical training on cardiovascular tissues. In terms of the respiratory system personal trainers should be familiar with breathing mechanics, aspects of gas exchange and the effects of smoking, which might play a role in the lifestyles of their clients.

Cardiovascular System

The cardiovascular system is a finely tuned system that transports oxygen and nutrients to the tissues where these are needed and removes metabolites and other waste products. A proper under-standing of this system is essential for the personal trainer to help customers with athletic performance, body recomposition, and gen-eral health.

Functional Anatomy of the Heart

In adults, the heart is about the size of a fist, and weighs between 250 and 350 grams. The human heart has four chambers: two atria (upper section) and two ventricles (lower section; see figure 8.1). The atria receive blood and the ventricles discharge it. Two circuits make up the route of blood through the human heart: the pulmonary circuit (deoxygenated blood) and the systemic circuit (oxygenated blood). In the pulmonary circuit deoxygenated blood passes through the

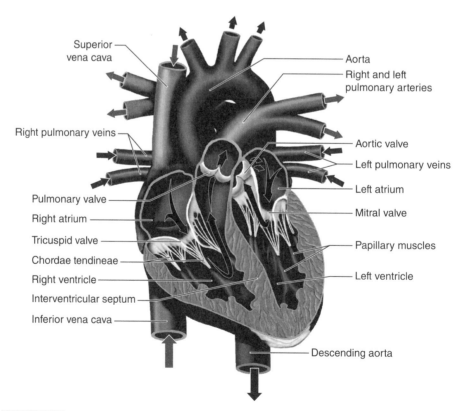

Figure 8.1 Anatomy of the heart.

superior vena cava and collects in the right atrium. Next the right atrium pumps the blood through the tricuspid valve into the right ventricle. From there the right ventricle pumps the blood through the pulmonary valve to the pulmonary arteries and into the lungs. In the systemic circuit oxygenated blood returns from the lungs through the pulmonary veins, coming first into the left atrium. The left atrium pumps the blood into the left ventricle through the mitral valve. Next the left ventricle pumps the blood through the aortic valve to the aorta. From there the blood moves to the rest of the body by means of the circulatory system (Standring 2008; Anderson et al. 2013).

The right side of the heart collects deoxygenated blood from the body in the right atrium. Next the atrium pumps this blood into the right ventricle, which pumps the blood again into the lungs. There the blood drops off carbon dioxide and picks up oxygen. While in the lungs the blood absorbs oxygen through a process of diffusion. At the same time oxygenated blood from the lungs moves into the left atrium. From the left atrium the blood passes through the bicuspid (or mitral) valve to the left ventricle, which pumps it out to the body via the aorta. Because of their function both ventricles are thicker and stronger than the atria. Because the left ventricle requires more force in order to pump the blood through the circulatory system to the rest of the body, its muscle wall is thicker than that of the right ventricle (Smith and Fernhall 2010).

Cardiac Cycle

Each heartbeat, also known as the cardiac cycle, involves a diastole and a systole. The diastole is the filling stage where blood moves from the atria into the ventricles. In the following stage, the systole, blood moves from the right ventricle to the pulmonary artery and from the left ventricle to the aorta. The aorta divides into major arteries, supplying blood to the upper and lower body. The blood travels through the arteries to smaller arterioles and then, finally, to tiny capillaries, supplying each cell with oxygen and nutrients. The deoxygenated blood passes to the venules, coalescing into veins, then to the inferior and superior venae cavae and once again back into the right atrium, thereby ending the cardiac cycle (Standring 2008).

Unlike skeletal muscles, which require either conscious or reflex nervous stimuli for excitation, cardiac muscles are self-exciting, receiving input from the sinus node with upwards of 100 beats per minute. Thus the heart's rhythmic contractions occur spontaneously, although nervous and hormonal factors, exercise and emotions all influence the rate of contraction. The sympathetic nervous system increases heart rate and the parasympathetic vagus nerve decreases heart rate (Klabunde 2011; Smith and Fernhall 2010).

Each heartbeat pumps out a certain volume of blood, or the stroke volume. The stroke volume at rest in the standing position averages between 60 and 80 millilitres of blood in most adults (see figure 8.2). The total volume of blood being pumped by the heart per minute is called the *cardiac output*, and it can be calculated as the product of stroke volume and heart rate.

Cardiac output = stroke volume × heart rate

At an average resting heart rate of 60 beats per minute cardiac output is approximately 5 litres per minute. Cardiac output adapts quickly to imposed demands, and it can increase severalfold through vigorous exercise. For example the cardiac output of Olympic medal winners in cross-country skiing increased eight times above resting cardiac output to approximately 40 litres per minute with an accompanying stroke volume of 210 millilitres per beat. For an average person maximal cardiac output during maximal leg or whole-body exercise is approximately 20 to 25 litres per minute. For all except the most trained endurance athletes, the limiting factor in aerobic capacity is cardiac output (Klabunde 2011; Smith and Fernhall 2010).

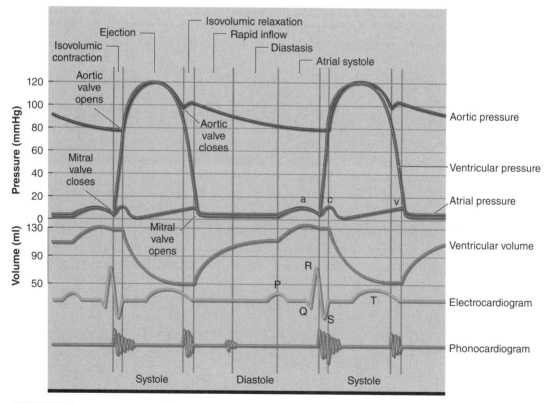

Figure 8.2   The cardiac cycle.

Reprinted, by permission, from W.L. Kenney, J.H. Wilmore, and D.L. Costill, 2015, *Physiology of sport and exercise,* 6th ed. (Champaign, IL: Human Kinetics), 161.

Blood Vessels

Blood travels though the body by means of the blood vessels. Three major types of blood vessels exist: the arteries, carrying blood from the heart to the organs; the capillaries, enabling exchange of water and nutrients between the blood and the tissues; and the veins, carrying blood from the capillaries back to the heart. The blood pressure in blood vessels is expressed in millimetres of mercury (1 mmHg = 133 pascals). In arteries the blood pressure at rest is approximately 120 mmHg systolic (high pressure wave due to contraction of the heart) and 80 mmHg diastolic (low pressure wave). On the other hand venous blood pressure is consistently low, usually staying under 10 mmHg. Superficial arteries can be located by feeling the heartbeat, for example, in the forearm and on the side of the neck. Vasoconstrictors control blood pressure by contracting the vascular smooth muscle in the vessel walls, thereby narrowing the vessels. Vasoconstrictors include paracrine factors (e.g., prostaglandins), hormones (e.g., vasopressin and angiotensin) and neurotransmitters (e.g., epinephrine). Vasodilation, or opening of blood vessels, is a similar process mediated by antagonistically acting mediators. Nitric oxide is the most prominent vasodilator in the human body (Klabunde 2011; Smith and Fernhall 2010).

Cardiovascular training causes new capillaries to be formed within the trained muscles, enabling transport of oxygen, carbon dioxide and other metabolites to and from the muscle fibres. Transportation of fatty acids from the bloodstream is upregulated through an increased number of transporter proteins within the walls of the blood vessels and in the muscle fibres. The increased number of capillaries together with increased fat transportation from the blood helps to improve the blood cholesterol profile.

Coronary Heart Disease

Coronary heart disease is one of the most common causes of death in the Western world. It kills every fourth adult in the United States alone. This affects both genders equally. Risk factors for coronary heart disease include physical inactivity, high blood pressure, smoking, high blood cholesterol, diabetes, family history, age, stress and obesity. A study from 2009 showed that low cardiorespiratory fitness (determined by a maximal exercise test on a treadmill) and hypertension are the two biggest risk factors for death in the Western world (Blair 2009). Making the following lifestyle changes can effectively reduce (or reverse, in the case of diet) coronary heart disease: choosing a healthy diet, controlling weight, quitting smoking, exercising and increasing intake of Omega-3 fatty acids (Pedersen and Saltin 2006).

Effects of Physical Training on Cardiovascular Tissues

Aerobic training increases the size of the ventricles, which allows the heart to pump more blood to the body. Resistance training thickens the myocardial wall; thus when the heart muscle contracts, more blood is pushed through the arteries compressed by the contraction. This thickening (or hypertrophy) is reversible and non-pathological. If the stress on the body from the resistance training is volume over-load (e.g., aerobic exercise increases return of blood to the heart), the sarcomeres in the ventricle muscle lengthen rather than thicken, dilating the ventricle (i.e., expanding the heart) and thus allowing a greater volume of blood flow to the heart. This process of thickening of the ventricular wall is called *eccentric hypertrophy*. The increase in thickness is proportional to the increase in the chamber's radius. The chamber radius might not change with pressure overload (e.g., resistance training compresses arteries and thus increases resistance to blood flow). The ventricular wall does, however, get much thicker as new sarcomeres are added in parallel to existing sarcomeres, a phenomenon called *concentric hypertrophy*. Ventricles with concentric hypertrophy can generate greater forces and higher pressures, whilst maintaining normal stress to the muscle wall.

Long-term effects of aerobic exercise on the heart include increased stroke volume and consequently lowered resting heart rate. Training increases the number of capillaries in the heart, thereby increasing blood supply to the heart's own muscles.

The net results of cardiovascular training are reduced risk of heart disease, reduction of high blood pressure and improved blood cholesterol (Klabunde 2011; Smith and Fernhall 2010).

Respiratory System

The respiratory system is the anatomical system that performs gas exchange. It includes the airways, lungs and the respiratory muscles (see figure 8.3). The gas exchange occurs in the alveoli of the lungs, where oxygen and carbon dioxide molecules diffuse passively between the gaseous external environment and the blood.

Breathing Mechanics

Breathing is an unconscious process. To meet the body's needs, specialised centres in the brainstem automatically regulate the rate and depth of breathing. The rate of respiration is higher during exercise, when aerobic metabolism in the muscles increases the level of

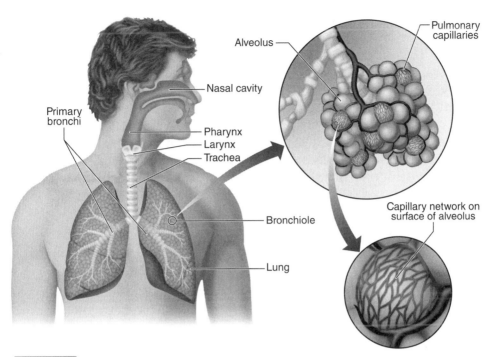

Pulmonary
capillaries

Alveolus

Nasal cavity

Primary
bronchi

Pharynx
Larynx
Trachea

Bronchiole

Capillary network on
surface of alveolus

Lung

Figure 8.3 Anatomy of the respiratory system.

carbon dioxide in the blood, which then activates carotid and aortic bodies in the respiration centre of the heart. Breathing rate is lower during rest because carbon dioxide level is also lower. Note that this buildup of carbon dioxide (not a lack of oxygen) is what leads to the feeling of being out of breath during exercise. This is because carbon dioxide levels during activity make the blood more acidic. The brain's automatic controls ensure that the muscles and other organs receive an appropriate amount of oxygen by increasing and then upregulating the rate and depth of ventilation.

Normally adults breathe 10 to 18 times per minute, with a breathing time of 2 seconds. During vigorous inhalation such as during exercise (at rates exceeding 35 breaths per minute), or in approaching respiratory failure, accessory muscles support respiration, including the sternocleidomastoid, platysma, scalene muscles of the neck, the pectoral muscles and the latissimus dorsi. The diaphragm initiates inhalation with support from the external intercostal muscles. The ribcage expands as the diaphragm contracts, pushing the contents of the abdomen downward, increasing thoracic volume and negative pressure inside the thorax and causing pressure in the chest to fall. As this happens air moves into the conducting zone in the lungs. Here it is filtered, warmed and humidified.

The accessory muscles and external intercostal muscles help the thoracic cavity expand even more during forced inhalation (e.g., during deep breathing). In contrast to the active contraction of the diaphragm during inhalation, exhalation generally happens passively. Nonetheless exhalation can also be forced (e.g., blowing out a candle). This happens with the help of the internal intercostal and abdominal muscles, which generate pressure in the thorax and abdomen to push air out of the lungs. Pulmonary ventilation is not a limiting factor for supplying the system with oxygen during exercise; consequently long-term exercise has little effect on the respiratory system. (Klabunde 2011; Smith and Fernhall 2010; Standring 2008).

Gas Exchange

As previously mentioned gas exchange (i.e., between the air we breathe and the circulatory system) occurs in the lungs. This exchange is the major function of the respiratory system, removing carbon dioxide and other gaseous metabolites from the blood that returns from the body through the veins and simultaneously supplying oxygen to the blood to be delivered to the body through the arteries. This process is made possible because of pressure difference (Klabunde 2011; Smith and Fernhall 2010).

The site of gas exchange is the alveoli, the basic functional unit of the lungs. These tiny sacs have extremely thin walls, approximately 1/5,000 of a millimetre, that are made up of a single layer of epithelial cells. The cells in the alveolar walls are close to the pulmonary capillaries, which are also made up of a single layer of cells (in this case, endothelial cells). Because these two types of cells are so close to one another, they are permeable to gases, thus allowing the gas exchange to occur.

Smoking and Pulmonary Function

Smoking has both acute and long-term negative effects on pulmonary function. Within seconds of inhalation of tobacco smoke, the airways narrow. This is regarded as a defensive lung reflex. During the first seconds after smoke inhalation, lung conductance may decrease as much as 40 percent in non-smokers; after 1 minute the conductance is decreased by approximately 15 percent (Rees et al. 1982).

Long-term cigarette smoking can both affect the immune system and induce pulmonary disorders such as chronic obstructive pulmonary disease (COPD), which is currently the fourth leading cause of chronic morbidity and mortality worldwide. The obstruction to airflow that develops in 15 to 20 percent of heavy smokers is thought to be due to abnormalities in airways with an internal diameter of less than

2 millimetres (Hogg et al. 2004). Previous studies from several laboratories have shown that this airway obstruction is associated with a chronic inflammatory process in the membranous and respiratory bronchioles. Accordingly the most significant risk factor associated with COPD is exposure to cigarette smoke.

Conclusion

Aerobic fitness, or cardiorespiratory fitness, refers to the body's ability (by means of the circulatory and respiratory systems) to deliver oxygen to the skeletal muscles during physical activity. Regular exercise leads to hypertrophy of the heart muscle, increasing the thickness of the muscle wall. This allows the heart to pump more blood with each stroke. Aerobic exercise also increases the number of small arteries (and thus the blood supply) in the skeletal muscles being worked by the training. Consequently exercise improves the cardiorespiratory system by increasing the amount of oxygen that is inhaled and distributed to body tissue.

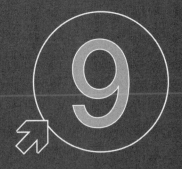

Nervous System

Alexis Batrakoulis

This chapter shows the role of the nervous system within the human body by presenting its basic structure and function and describing how it responds and adapts to exercise. Personal trainers must have a good knowledge of the anatomy and functionality of the nervous system in order to support and enhance their clients' performance and prevent injury because this system is responsible for the recruitment of muscles and learning of movement patterns.

The *nervous system* controls and co-ordinates the functioning of all other systems in response to our surroundings. Each stimulus or change in our environment is detected by our senses. Messages are interpreted by the brain, which in turn sends directions to the various organs to respond and adapt according to the external conditions that affect our body. Because all the major components of the human movement system affect each other, the nervous system must work with the skeletal and muscular systems to produce optimal movement (Clark et al. 2012). The nervous system is one of the major control systems contained within the human body; as such its function is to transmit and receive a constant series of messages via electrical impulses to and from the control centre situated in the brain (Tortora 2001).

Organisation of the Nervous System

In order to control movements, the body must be aware of how much force each muscle is generating. The nervous system provides information for modulating muscle actions. It is divided into two divisions:

- Central nervous system
- Peripheral nervous system

The *central nervous system* is composed of the brain and spinal cord. Its main function is to co-ordinate the activity of all parts of the body. This system receives input about the state of both the external and internal environments from the sense organs and receptors, which monitor events in and outside the body (Noback et al. 2005). Furthermore it collates all of the information, analyses the data (interpretation) and finally sends out messages in response to incoming data (motor output) via the motor neurons of the *peripheral nervous system* to the effectors (muscles and glands).

The *peripheral nervous system* contains only nerves (cranial and spine). It connects the brain and spinal cord to the rest of the body. These nerves are divided into sensory nerves, which conduct messages from various parts of the body to the central nervous system, and motor nerves, which conduct impulses from the central nervous system to the muscles and glands (figure 9.1).

The peripheral nervous system is further divided into the following systems:

- Somatic nervous system
- Autonomic nervous system

The *somatic nervous system* consists of sensory neurons from the head, body wall, extremities and motor neurons. It conveys information from the central nervous system efferently to skeletal muscle, ultimately leading to muscle contraction. The motor responses are under conscious control, and therefore the somatic nervous system is voluntary (Noback et al. 2005).

The *autonomic nervous system* consists of nerves that supply neural input to the involuntary systems of the body, such as cardiac muscle, smooth muscle in the walls of the digestive system, endocrine glands and other tissues and organs (Fox 2006). In addition the autonomic nervous system is divided into two parts:

- Sympathetic nervous system
- Parasympathetic nervous system

These two systems provide nerve stimuli to the same organs throughout the body, but bring about different effects. Both of them are

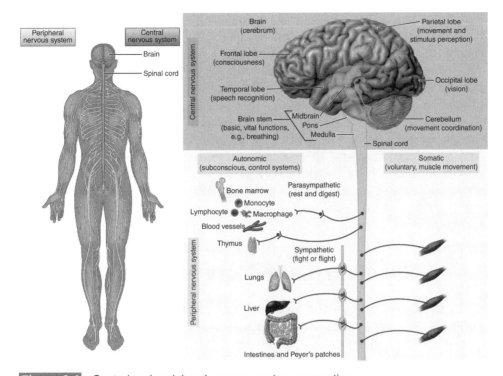

Figure 9.1 Central and peripheral nervous system connections.

From Robbins, D., and E. Zeinstra. 2015. Muscle action. In *Europe Active's Foundations for Exercise Professionals,* edited by T. Rieger, F. Naclerio, A. Jiménez, and J. Moody. Champaign, IL: Human Kinetics.

essential for preparing the body for the stress of exercise and returning the body back to normal conditions (figure 9.2). Specifically, the *sympathetic nervous system* helps prepare the body for fight or flight and creates conditions in the tissues for physical activity. It is stimulated by strong emotions such as anger and excitement, speeding up heart rate, increasing the activity of sweat glands and adrenal glands, and decreasing activity in the digestive system. It also produces rapid redistribution of blood between the skin and skeletal muscles. In

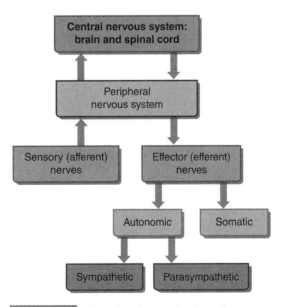

Figure 9.2 Functional organisation of nervous system.

Reprinted, by permission, from W.L. Kenney, J.H. Wilmore, and D.L. Costill, 2015, *Physiology of sport and exercise,* 6th ed. (Champaign, IL: Human Kinetics), 74.

general it helps the body prepare for activity, speeding up responses (e.g., increasing heart rate) and mobilising energy stores to get us ready for action (Noback et al. 2005).

In contrast the *parasympathetic nervous system* slows down the body and helps it prepare for a more relaxed state, such as for digestion and sleep. It increases peristalsis of the alimentary canal, slows down the heart rate and constricts the bronchioles in the lungs. In general it decreases the body's levels of activation during rest and recovery, and it is more active during periods of calm and relaxation. The balance between these two systems is controlled to create a state of homeostasis, that is, where the internal stability of the bodily systems is maintained in response to the external environment (Fox 2006).

Function of the Nervous System

The functional unit of the nervous system is the neuron. This specialised cell processes and transmits information through both electrical and chemical signals (figure 9.3). Neurons are composed of three main parts: the cell body, axon and dendrites. The cell body

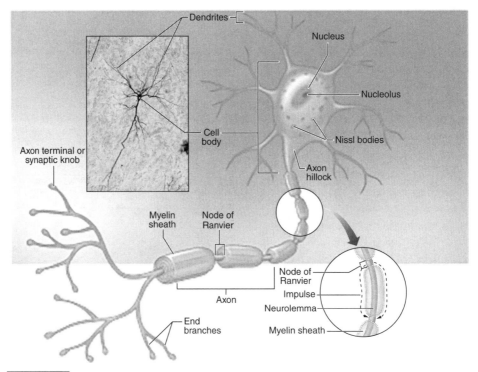

Figure 9.3   The neuron.

From Lodish, H., A. Berk, S.L. Zipursky et al. 2000. *Molecular Cell Biology*. 4th ed. New York: W.H. Freeman.

(or soma) of a neuron contains a nucleus and other organelles, including lysosomes, mitochondria and a Golgi complex. The axon is a cylindrical projection from the cell body that transmits nervous impulses to other neurons or effector sites (muscles, organs). The axon is the part of the neuron that provides communication from the brain and spinal cord to other parts of the body. The dendrites gather information from other structures and transmit it back to the neuron (Tortora 2001).

As the functional units of this system, neurons are divided into three categories in accordance of their functionality (Vander et al. 2001):

- Sensory neurons
- Interneurons
- Motor neurons

Sensory neurons respond to touch, sound, light and other stimuli and transmit nerve impulses from muscles and organs to the brain and spinal cord. *Interneurons* transmit nerve impulses from one neuron to another. *Motor neurons* transmit nerve impulses from the brain and spinal cord to the muscles or glands (Noback et al. 2005).

The main responsibilities of the nervous system include three primary functions (figure 9.4):

- Sensory function
- Integrative function
- Motor function

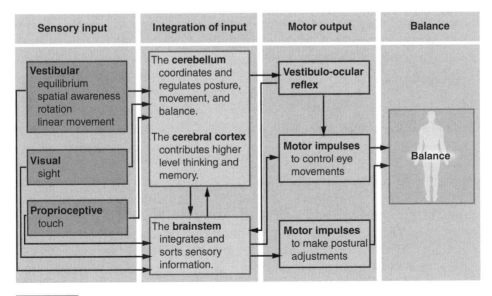

Figure 9.4 Functionality of neurons.
Based on Hanes and McCollum 2006.

Sensory function is the ability of the nervous system to detect various stimuli by monitoring events inside (e.g., muscle stretch or contraction) or outside the human body (e.g., specific surface, environmental temperature). Information is then conveyed afferently to the central nervous system.

Integrative function is the ability of the nervous system to analyse and interpret the sensory information, allowing for proper decision making, or producing an appropriate response to stimuli.

Motor function is the body's neuromuscular response to the incoming data (sensory information).

Sensory receptors are located throughout the body. They are divided into four categories:

- Mechanoreceptors
- Nociceptors
- Chemoreceptors
- Photoreceptors

Mechanoreceptors respond to mechanical forces (e.g., touch and pressure), *nociceptors* respond to pain, *chemoreceptors* respond to chemical interaction (e.g., smell and taste) and, finally, *photoreceptors* respond to light (e.g., vision).

The most familiar category of these receptors with regard to human movement are *mechanoreceptors*, specialised structures that respond to mechanical pressure within tissues and provide information about pressure, length, tension, position and motion to the central nervous system (Clark et al. 2012). These receptors are located in muscles, tendons, ligaments, joints and skin. They have three components:

- Muscle spindles
- Golgi tendon organs
- Joint receptors

Muscle spindles are sensory stretch receptors (proprioceptors) in the belly of a muscle, running parallel to the muscle fibres (Hoffman 2002). They primarily detect changes in length of the muscle, as well as the rate of change in length, and convey information to the central nervous system regarding static changes in muscle length or joint angle. The coiled nerves stretch as the muscles stretch, sending information back to the central nervous system about the relative length of the muscle (figure 9.5). These receptors enhance human performance. They are critical because they initiate the *stretch reflex*, a monosynaptic reflex where muscle force production is enhanced when the muscle is previously stretched. A reflex itself is an involuntary response. It reflects a time component because more force is pro-

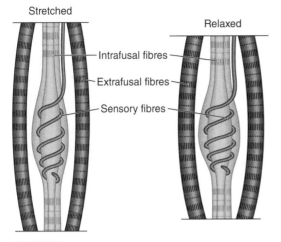

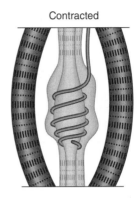

Figure 9.5 Muscle spindles.

duced in a short period of time. When a muscle is stretched, information is sent from the muscle spindles to the spinal cord, where a potent muscular response ensues. The stretch reflex enhances muscular performance and efficiency, and it is trainable (Baechle and Earle 2008).

Another form of neural feedback is from a special sensory receptor found in the tendons called the *Golgi tendon organ* (McArdle et al. 2005). This receptor is a proprioceptive sensory compo-

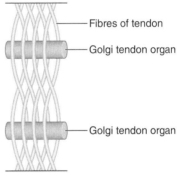

Figure 9.6 Golgi tendon organs.

nent that is woven into the fibres of tendons (figure 9.6). Due to its location, its primary role is to convey information regarding muscle tension to the central nervous system. Specifically, as muscle tension increases, so does the amount of stretch in the Golgi tendon organ. Once a threshold level of tension is attained, its activity increases greatly. The Golgi tendon organ responds by causing agonist muscle relaxation and antagonist muscle excitation. It protects the body from excessive damage (Ratamess 2012).

The final type of receptor considered here is the *joint receptor*. Joint receptors are located in and around the joints. They respond to pressure and acceleration and deceleration of the joint. Joint receptors provide awareness of position, rather than muscle length and tension, like the muscle spindles and Golgi tendon organs do. These receptors signal extreme joint positions, and thus help prevent injury. They can also initiate a reflexive inhibitory response in the surrounding muscles if too much stress is placed on that joint (Fox 2006).

At this point of the chapter, we must define proprioception and the role of proprioceptors in human movement. *Proprioception* is the cumulative sensory input to the central nervous system from all the mechanoreceptors that sense body position and limb movement. A general way to think about it is the body's ability to sense the relative position of its adjacent parts. The *proprioceptors* are specialised sensory receptors that provide the central nervous system with information needed to maintain muscle tone and perform complex co-ordinated movements. Increasing of proprioception through balance training will enhance muscular performance and many motor skills and help prevent injuries (Drury 2000; Grigg 1994; Lephart et al. 1997). Thus, personal trainers must know how to train the nervous system in order to ensure safety and help their clients obtain optimal results.

Nervous System and Exercise

The nervous system can be trained and improved with repetitive exercises in order to enhance the motor skills of co-ordination and balance. Personal trainers can help their clients progressively attempt, practise and perfect new and extended movements involving musculoskeletal action. They can also help clients focus on using the voluntary nervous system to initiate those actions. The nervous system is adversely affected by age. As we grow older neurons are lost and are not replaced. The nervous system's capacity to transmit impulses to and from the brain decreases, and both voluntary and reflex actions become slower. Beginning clients improve their performance because they make many changes to the way the central nervous system controls and co-ordinates movement. This is more common in resistance training; thus systematic practice causes adaptations in the central nervous system, allowing for greater control of movement, more accuracy and higher performance. Exercise training may elicit adaptations along the neuromuscular chain, starting in the higher brain centres and continuing down to the level of individual muscle fibres (Brooks et al. 2008).

In general these adaptations are important for increased co-ordination, strength, power, speed, motor-unit recruitment, firing rates, synchronisation and reflex potentiation, as well as decreased Golgi tendon organ sensitivity. Potentiation involves the creation of a set of stimulatory circumstances within the muscle firing complex that boosts neural excitation and motor-unit and muscle-fibre recruitment and reduces inhibition (Baechle and Earle 2008). However any potentiating activity must not fatigue the central nervous system; otherwise the reverse effect will be experienced. Especially in case of resistance training, when the priority is the enhancement of muscular strength or power, trainers must focus on the quality of execution of an exercise rather than the quantity of repetitions (Ratamess 2012).

One last important element concerning the effectiveness of nervous system training is appropriate programming in order to ensure optimal recovery between workouts, especially when the anaerobic system (strength, power and speed training) is used intensively and frequently (Bompa and Carrera 2005).

Conclusion

Professional personal trainers must have adequate knowledge of the nervous system and its anatomy and physiology in order to understand the scientific basis for human movement. The nervous system and two others (skeletal and muscular) are linked as a kinetic chain that produces motion. It is composed of billions of neurons that transfer information throughout the body. Its function is to transmit and receive a constant series of messages via electrical impulses to and from the control centre situated in the brain. The knowledge and understanding of this information is absolutely crucial for developing exercise programmes that meet the individualised needs and priorities of clients according to the neuromuscular aspects of physical activity (Gardiner 2001).

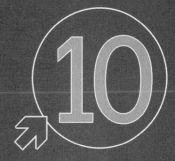

Hormonal Responses to Exercise

Sabrena Merrill
Cedric X. Bryant

The *endocrine system,* which is made up of various glands through-out the body, is responsible for regulating bodily activities through the production of hormones. Hormones regulate growth, metabolism, sexual development and function, and responses to stress. Because of their involvement in the regulation of metabolism, hormones play a significant role in the body's responses to acute exercise and chronic physical training.

Structural Overview of the Endocrine System

Located throughout the body are the different endocrine glands: pituitary, thyroid, parathyroid, adrenal, pineal and thymus. In addition to glands specifically designed for endocrine function, discrete areas within certain tissues also produce hormones: in the pancreas, gonads and hypothalamus. Having no ducts endocrine glands release their hormones directly into the extracellular spaces around the tissues, where the hormones diffuse into the bloodstream for transport to *target organs.* In contrast other types of structures, called *exocrine glands,* release their secretions from ducts that carry substances directly to a specific area or surface. Examples of exocrine glands include sweat and saliva glands.

Pituitary Gland

The *pituitary gland* is often referred to as the master gland because of its regulatory effect on several other endocrine glands and its importance in controlling a number of diverse bodily functions. No larger than a pea the pituitary gland is located at the base of the brain beneath the *hypothalamus* and is divided into anterior and posterior lobes (see figure 10.1).

The posterior lobe releases a hormone called *vasopressin* or *antidiuretic hormone* (*ADH*). It acts on the kidneys, and is considered an *antidiuretic* (i.e., a substance that inhibits urine production, thereby aiding in the retention of bodily fluid). ADH, in essence, controls water loss by the kidneys. The posterior portion also releases *oxytocin*, a hormone that stimulates the smooth muscles of the reproductive organs and intestines. In women, oxytocin contracts the uterus during childbirth and stimulates breast-milk production. The hormones secreted by the posterior pituitary are actually produced in the hypothalamus and carried to the pituitary gland through nerves.

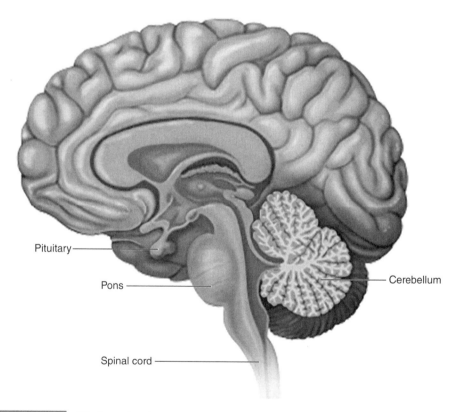

Pituitary

Pons

Cerebellum

Spinal cord

Figure 10.1 Pituitary gland.

Thus these hormones are essentially stored in the pituitary gland and released as needed through neural stimulation.

The anterior portion of the pituitary gland releases six hormones that affect various important bodily functions: *follicle-stimulating hormone (FSH), luteinising hormone (LH), thyroid-stimulating hormone (TSH), adrenocorticotropin hormone (ACTH), growth hormone (GH),* and *prolactin.* FSH and LH are called *gonadotropins* because of their effects on the gonads (ovaries and testes). These substances control the secretion of *oestrogen* and *progesterone* in the ovaries and the production of *testosterone* in the testicles. TSH stimulates the synthesis and release of *thyroxine (T_4)* from the *thyroid gland,* which helps control the rate at which all cells use oxygen. ACTH controls the secretion in the *adrenal gland* of hormones that influence the metabolism of carbohydrate, sodium and potassium. ACTH also controls the rate at which substances are exchanged between the blood and tissues. GH stimulates growth in general and specifically of the skeletal system. Additionally GH promotes the entrance of *amino acids* into the body's cells for their incorporation into protein and releases fatty acids into the blood for use as energy. GH has also been shown to promote the formation of glucose and its release into the blood. Lastly prolactin is involved in the initiation and maintenance of breast-milk production and secretion in women.

Thyroid Gland

The thyroid gland is a butterfly-shaped structure located anterior to the upper part of the trachea, and is among the largest endocrine organs in the body (see figure 10.2). Mentioned earlier for its functions controlled by the pituitary gland, the thyroid gland releases three hormones: T_4, *triiodothyronine (T_3)* and *calcitonin.*

Often called the major metabolic hormones, T_4 and T_3 are iodine-containing hormones that are released by the thyroid to regulate the metabolism of carbohydrate, protein and lipids, thereby increasing the body's oxygen consumption and heat production. These hormones also work to maintain blood pressure by causing an increase in adrenergic receptors in blood vessels, thus facilitating *vasoconstriction.*

The third hormone, calcitonin, lowers blood calcium and phosphate levels by accelerating the absorption of calcium by the bones. The skeleton is in a constant state of remodelling whereby old bone is cleaved away by cells called *osteoclasts* and new bone is laid down by cells called *osteoblasts.* Calcitonin inhibits bone removal by the osteoclasts whilst simultaneously promoting bone formation by the osteoblasts.

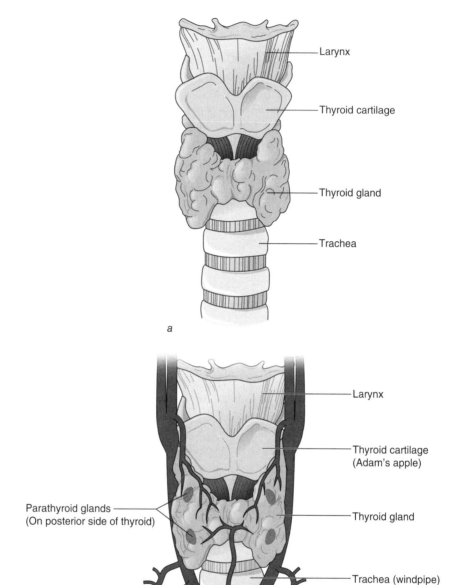

Figure 10.2 (a) Thyroid gland and (b) parathyroid glands.

Parathyroid Glands

The parathyroid glands consist of four structures—sometimes more depending on a person's anatomy—located on the posterior surface of the thyroid gland. These glands release parathyroid hormone (PTH), which is primarily responsible for controlling the levels of calcium and phosphorus in the blood through its actions on the kidneys, skeleton and small intestine. When blood calcium levels are low PTH increases bone *resorption* (i.e., stimulates osteoclasts), breaking down bone calcium for its release into the blood. PTH also signals the kidneys to reabsorb calcium so that it is not lost in the urine, and provokes increased calcium absorption by the intestinal wall. Furthermore PTH works synergistically with vitamin D to maintain the body's calcium levels.

Adrenal Glands

The adrenal glands appear as two pyramid-shaped organs located close to the superior border of each kidney. Each gland consists of two distinct parts: the medulla (inner portion) and the cortex (outer portion). The adrenal medulla and the adrenal cortex are so distinct that each portion is, in effect, its own distinct endocrine organ. The adrenal medulla is part of the sympathetic nervous system and produces two hormones: *epinephrine* (adrenaline) and *norepinephrine* (noradrenaline). Collectively these substances are called *catecholamines*, and they function co-operatively to prepare the body for emergencies or stressful events.

Epinephrine acts to elevate blood glucose levels; increase the rate, force and amplitude of the heartbeat; and dilate blood vessels that feed the heart, lungs and skeletal muscles. The release of norepinephrine causes an increase in heart rate and in the force of contraction of the cardiac muscle. It also contributes to constriction of blood vessels in most areas of the body. The adrenal cortex secretes *mineralocorticoids* associated with the metabolism of the mineral salts sodium and potassium, *glucocorticoids* that aid in the utilisation of glucose and mobilisation of fatty acids, and a small amount of *gonadocorticoids*, including testosterone, oestrogen and progesterone.

Pancreas

The pancreas is situated behind and slightly below the stomach. In addition to its role in producing digestive enzymes (an exocrine function) it serves as an endocrine gland that produces hormones involved in regulating carbohydrate metabolism (see figure 10.3). Structures called the islets of Langerhans within the pancreas contain *alpha cells* (α-cells) and *beta cells* (β-cells).

The β-cells secrete *insulin*, which acts to facilitate the uptake and utilisation of glucose (blood sugar) by cells and prevent the breakdown of *glycogen* (the storage form of glucose) in the liver and muscle. This function makes insulin a powerful hypoglycaemic agent—that is, it decreases the blood sugar level. Insulin also plays a role in

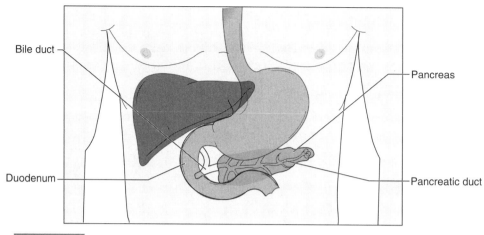

Figure 10.3 Pancreas.

lipid and protein metabolism because it favours lipid formation and storage and facilitates the movement of amino acids into cells. The α-cells secrete *glucagon*, which generally opposes the actions of insulin. Glucagon decreases glucose oxidation and increases the blood sugar level (hyperglycaemia). Its main action appears to be stimulation of the breakdown of glycogen in the liver for its release into the bloodstream.

Gonads

The gonads are the endocrine glands that produce hormones that promote sex-specific physical characteristics and regulate reproductive function. The sex hormones testosterone and oestrogen are found in both males and females, but in varying concentrations. In males, testosterone is produced in the testes and acts to initiate sperm production, stimulate the development of male secondary sex characteristics and promote tissue building. Testosterone's *anabolic* (tissue-building) function contributes to the male–female differences in muscle mass and strength that first appear during puberty. In females, the ovaries are the primary source for the production of oestrogens, which include *estradiol* and progesterone. Oestrogens regulate ovulation, menstruation, physiological adjustments during pregnancy and the appearance of female secondary sex characteristics. Furthermore oestrogen affects the blood vessels, bones, lungs, liver, intestines, prostate and testes. Table 10.1 lists the major endocrine glands and summarises some selected effects of their associated hormones.

Table 10.1 The Major Endocrine Glands and Their Hormones, Target Organs, Controlling Factors and Functions

Endocrine gland	Hormone	Target organ	Controlling factor	Major functions
Anterior pituitary	Growth hormone (GH)	All cells in the body	Hypothalamic GH-releasing hormone; GH-inhibiting hormone (somatostatin)	Promotes development and enlargement of all body tissues until maturation; increases rate of protein synthesis; increases mobilization of fats and use of fat as an energy source; decreases rate of carbohydrate use
	Thyrotropin (TSH)	Thyroid gland	Hypothalamic TSH-releasing hormone	Controls the amount of thyroxin and triiodothyronine produced and released by the thyroid gland
	Adrenocorticotropin (ACTH)	Adrenal cortex	Hypothalamic ACTH-releasing hormone	Controls the secretion of hormones from the adrenal cortex
	Prolactin	Breasts	Prolactin-releasing and -inhibiting hormones	Stimulates milk production by the breasts
	Follicle-stimulating hormone (FSH)	Ovaries, testes	Hypothalamic FSH-releasing hormone	Initiates growth of follicles in the ovaries and promotes secretion of estrogen from the ovaries; promotes development of the sperm in the testes
	Luteinizing hormone (LH)	Ovaries, testes	Hypothalamic FSH-releasing hormone	Promotes secretion of estrogen and progesterone and causes the follicle to rupture, releasing the ovum; causes testes to secrete testosterone
Posterior pituitary	Antidiuretic hormone (ADH or vasopressin)	Kidneys	Hypothalamic secretory neurons	Assists in controlling water excretion by the kidneys; elevates blood pressure by constricting blood vessels
	Oxytocin	Uterus, breasts	Hypothalamic secretory neurons	Controls contraction of uterus; milk secretion
Thyroid	Thyroxine (T4) and triiodothyronine (T3)	All cells in the body	TSH, T3, and T4 concentrations	Increase the rate of cellular metabolism; increase rate and contractility of the heart
	Calcitonin	Bones	Plasma calcium concentrations	Controls calcium ion concentration in the blood

(continued)

Table 10.1 *(continued)*

Endocrine gland	Hormone	Target organ	Controlling factor	Major functions
Parathyroid	Parathyroid hormone (PTH or parathormone)	Bones, intestines, and kidneys	Plasma calcium concentrations	Controls calcium ion concentration in the extracellular fluid through its influence on bones, intestines, and kidneys
Adrenal medulla	Epinephrine	Most cells in the body	Baroreceptors, glucose receptors, brain and spinal centers	Stimulates breakdown of glycogen in liver and muscle and lipolysis in adipose tissue and muscle; increases skeletal muscle blood flow; increases heart rate and contractility; increases oxygen consumption
	Norepinephrine	Most cells in the body	Baroreceptors, glucose receptors, brain and spinal centers	Stimulates lipolysis in adipose tissue and in muscle to a lesser extent; constricts arterioles and venules, thereby elevating blood pressure
Adrenal cortex	Mineralocorticoids (aldosterone)	Kidneys	Angiotensin and plasma potassium concentrations; renin	Increase sodium retention and potassium excretion through the kidneys
	Glucocorticoids (cortisol)	Most cells in the body	ACTH	Control metabolism of carbohydrates, fats, and proteins; exert an anti-inflammatory action
	Androgens and estrogens	Ovaries, breasts, and testes	ACTH	Assist in the development of female and male sex characteristics
Pancreas	Insulin	All cells in the body	Plasma glucose and amino acid concentrations	Controls blood glucose levels by lowering glucose levels; increases use of glucose and synthesis of fat
	Glucagon	All cells in the body	Plasma glucose and amino acid concentrations	Increases blood glucose; stimulates the breakdown of protein and fat
	Somatostatin	Islets of Langerhans and intestines	Plasma glucose, insulin, and glucagon concentrations	Depresses the secretion of both insulin and glucagon
Kidney	Renin	Adrenal cortex	Plasma sodium concentrations	Assists in blood pressure control
	Erythropoietin (EPO)	Bone marrow	Low tissue oxygen concentrations	Stimulates erythrocyte production

Endocrine gland	Hormone	Target organ	Controlling factor	Major functions
Testes	Testosterone	Sex organs, muscle	FSH and LH	Promotes development of male sex characteristics, including growth of testes, scrotum, and penis, facial hair, and change in voice; also promotes muscle growth
Ovaries	Ostrogens and progesterone	Sex organs and adipose tissue	FSH and LH	Promote development of female sex organs and characteristics; increase storage of fat; assist in regulating the menstrual cycle

Reprinted, by permission, from W.L. Kenney, J.H. Wilmore, and D.L. Costill, 2015, *Physiology of sport and exercise*, 6th ed. (Champaign, IL: Human Kinetics), 102.

Classification of Hormones

Hormones are chemical substances produced by endocrine tissues that generally fit into one of two categories: steroid-derived hormones and hormones synthesised from protein. The chemical make-up of hormones determines how they interact with target sites throughout the body. Most *steroid* hormones are manufactured from *cholesterol*, which makes them soluble in lipids and allows them to diffuse rather easily through cell membranes. The adrenal cortex, ovaries, testes and placenta secrete steroid hormones (table 10.2). Non-steroid hormones are subdivided further into those made from protein, or *peptide* hormones, and those produced from amino acids. This group of hormones is soluble in blood plasma, but they cannot cross the cell membrane so they must interact with specialised receptors on the outside of the cell, on the cell membrane. The thyroid gland and adrenal medulla secrete amino acid hormones (table 10.2), whereas all other non-steroid hormones are made from protein or peptide hormones.

Substances called *prostaglandins* are often considered to be a third class of hormones, although technically they are not. Prostaglandins are biologically active lipids found in the plasma membrane of most cells. Typically prostaglandins act as local hormones, meaning that they exert their effects on the immediate area where they are produced and released. However some can remain intact long enough to circulate in the bloodstream and affect other more distant tissues. Prostaglandins have many functions, but the function most related to the scope of this chapter is their action on blood vessels. Prostaglandins are important mediators of the inflammation response because they increase vascular permeability (which promotes swelling) and *vasodilation*. In addition they sensitise nerve

Table 10.2　Major Endocrine Organs and the Types of Hormones They Produce

Endocrine organ	Type of hormone produced
Steroid hormones	
Adrenal cortex	Cortisol and aldosterone
Ovaries	Oestrogen and progesterone
Testes	Testosterone
Placenta	Oestrogen and progesterone
Non-steroid hormones	
Thyroid	Thyroxine and triiodothyronine
Adrenal medulla	Epinephrine and norepinephrine
Pancreas	Insulin and glucagon
Anterior pituitary	Growth hormone, gonadotropins, thyroid stimulating hormone, adrenocorticotropin hormone and prolactin

endings of pain receptors, making prostaglandins a contributor to both inflammation and pain.

Hormone Interactions With Target Cells

When hormones are released into the bloodstream, they are carried to a specific organ or tissue containing target cells where they can perform their intended functions. Hormones can affect the target cells in one of four ways:

- Modify cellular protein synthesis
- Alter the rate of cellular enzyme activity
- Change plasma membrane permeability
- Promote secretory activity

The target cell's ability to respond to the influence of a hormone depends on the number of target cell receptors that occur either on the cell's membrane (for non-steroid hormones) or within the cell's interior (for steroid hormones). Hormones connect with their appropriate target cells through a lock-and-key arrangement in which the lock (receptor) can only be opened by a specific key (hormone).

Cells typically have 2,000 to 10,000 hormone receptors. However, the number of receptors can be altered to increase or decrease the cell's sensitivity to the hormone based on physiologic demand. A process called *downregulation* occurs when an increased amount of a specific hormone decreases the number of receptors available to it, making the cell less sensitive to the hormone. This occurs as a physiological mechanism to prevent target cells from over-responding to persistently high hormone levels. Downregulation can be seen in people with obesity, since they appear to have a reduction in the number of cells responsive to insulin. Due to the elevated levels of blood glucose in an obese person, the β-cells in the pancreas must release more insulin than usual to meet the demand and return the blood to homeostatic levels. This near-constant increase in blood insulin levels can cause target cells on the liver to downregulate and decrease the number of receptors for insulin, increasing the subject's resistance by decreasing sensitivity to this hormone. Obese people with chronic insulin resistance (or insulin insensitivity) are at risk for developing type 2 diabetes.

In contrast, *upregulation* describes a state in which target cells develop a greater number of receptors in response to increasing hormone levels. Upregulation is not as common in human physiology, but it does occur. An example of upregulation can be seen during the third trimester of pregnancy when there is an increase in uterine oxytocin receptors, which ultimately promotes the contraction of the uterus during childbirth.

Steroid Hormone Activity

Because steroid hormones are lipid based, they pass easily through the cell membrane. Once inside the cell steroid hormones bind with specific receptors, forming a hormone-receptor complex that then enters the cell's nucleus and binds with the cell's *deoxyribonucleic acid (DNA)* to activate certain genes. This process is called *direct gene activation*, and it causes *messenger ribonucleic acid (mRNA)* to be synthesised within the nucleus. The mRNA is the template for protein synthesis, since it carries instructions from the nucleus to the cytoplasm to manufacture new proteins (see figure 10.4). These proteins may be used for creating enzymes that affect cellular processes, developing structural proteins to be used for tissue growth or repair or making regulatory proteins that can change enzymatic function.

Non-steroid Hormone Activity

Non-steroid hormones cannot cross the cell membrane, so they must interact with specific receptors on the cell membrane. Thus it takes two sets of messengers to deliver the signals required to carry out the intended action of the hormone. Once a non-steroid hormone

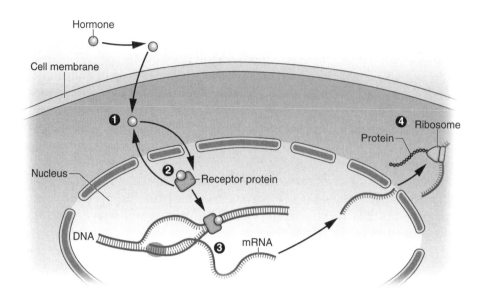

Figure 10.4 Steroid hormone action resulting in direct gene activation.

binds with its receptor, it triggers a sequence of enzymatic reactions that leads to the creation of a *second messenger*, which is a molecule inside the cell that transmits signals from the *first messenger* (hormone) to the target cell. A pervasive second messenger in the body called *cyclic adenosine monophosphate (cAMP)* activates an enzyme, adenylate cyclase, located within the cell membrane. This enzyme is relevant to physical exertion because it catalyses the formation of cAMP from cellular *adenosine triphosphate (ATP)*, which is the form of energy used by muscle cells to produce contractions (see figure 10.5). Another example of cAMP's role in an important physiological function is its contribution to bone and muscle growth and repair. The cAMP produced via growth hormone binding on muscle and bone cell membranes activates anabolic reactions to synthesise amino acids into tissue proteins.

Besides altering enzyme activity, non-steroid hormones can either facilitate or inhibit the uptake of certain substances by the cells. For example, insulin facilitates glucose transport into the cell. In contrast epinephrine inhibits insulin release, thereby slowing glucose uptake by the cells. Hormones can also exert both direct and indirect cellular effects. For example, insulin release prompts muscle fibres to take up glucose, which is a primary effect. In conjunction with glucose uptake, muscle fibres increase the synthesis of glycogen, which is

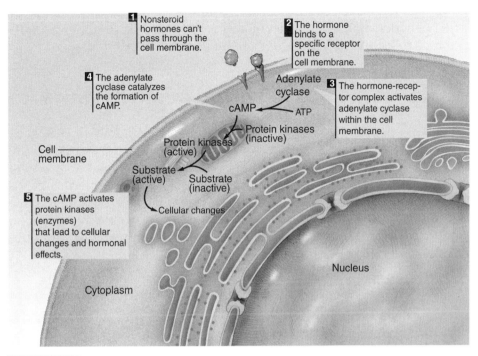

Figure 10.5 Non-steroid hormone action with an intracellular second messenger.

a secondary effect. Together these primary and secondary insulin effects work to maintain fuel *homeostasis* during a bout of exercise.

Negative Feedback System

Hormones are not released in a constant, steady stream, but rather are secreted in fluctuation depending on the physiologic demand for their actions. A *negative feedback system* is used to regulate the secretion of most hormones such that the release of a specific hormone is increased or decreased in response to physiologic changes. Some hormones are released in short bursts in periods of an hour or less, whilst others fluctuate over longer periods, showing daily or even monthly cycles (e.g., menstrual cycles).

The regulation of plasma glucose concentration is an example of how the endocrine system uses negative feedback to maintain homeostasis. When plasma glucose concentration is high, insulin is released by the pancreas in response to the negative feedback of elevated blood glucose levels. In response to insulin, cells take up glucose, thereby returning plasma glucose concentration to normal. Insulin release is then inhibited until plasma glucose levels rise again.

Thus, the negative feedback system alerts the brain to a stimulus, which in turn provokes a hormonal response that leads to an outcome of reducing or getting rid of the negative feedback.

Hormonal Responses to Acute Exercise

Up to this point, the discussion has focused primarily on the general structure and function of the endocrine system. Normal bodily function depends on the timely release and inhibition of a variety of hormones as they work together to bring about important actions at their target organs. The endocrine system plays a significant role in controlling physiological functions during exercise as well. The significant hormonal actions that are most responsive to an acute bout of exercise are presented in this section.

Anterior Pituitary Hormones

Working together with the hypothalamus, the anterior lobe of the pituitary gland has a widespread influence throughout the body. As noted earlier the hormones released by the anterior pituitary lobe are FSH, LH, TSH, ACTH, GH and prolactin. Of these six hormones, four are *tropic hormones* (i.e., FSH, LH, TSH and ACTH) and the remaining two (i.e., GH and prolactin) are non-tropic. Tropic hormones are substances that stimulate other endocrine organs to secrete their own hormones. For example, TSH stimulates the thyroid to release T_4. Once released T_4 circulates in the blood and stimulates metabolism in many types of cells. *Non-tropic hormones*, such as T_4, stimulate cellular growth, metabolism or other functions. GH is another example of a non-tropic hormone. Its functions include promoting muscle growth and *hypertrophy* and stimulating fat metabolism.

The hypothalamus is linked to the anterior pituitary lobe through a specialised circulatory system, which functions to transport specific hormones called *releasing factors* and *inhibiting factors* from the hypothalamus to the anterior pituitary lobe. Releasing factors are hormones that control the release of other hormones by stimulating the pituitary. That is, prior to the release of an anterior pituitary hormone, the anterior pituitary must be stimulated by the hypothalamus. Input from the nervous system about stimuli such as anxiety, stress and physical exertion controls the output of releasing factors from the hypothalamus. Inhibiting factors perform the opposite function by inhibiting pituitary hormone release. Thus although the pituitary gland has been called the master gland, it is really the hypothalamus that is controlling its functions.

Exercise provides a significant stimulus to the hypothalamus because it increases the release rate of all six anterior pituitary hormones. In particular GH concentrations are elevated during cardiorespiratory exercise in proportion to the exercise intensity, and they can remain elevated for a period of time after the activity ceases.

Growth Hormone

Because it promotes cell division and cellular proliferation throughout the body, GH plays a major role in protein synthesis. By facilitating amino acid transport through the cell membrane into the cells, GH acts as a potent anabolic agent. GH also supports the action of cortisol by decreasing glucose uptake by the tissues, increasing *free fatty acid* (FFA) mobilisation, and enhancing *gluconeogenesis* in the liver. The net effect of these actions is to preserve blood glucose concentration for use by the nervous system and muscle cells, thus augmenting performance during prolonged exercise.

Short-term physical activity (i.e., exercising to exhaustion) stimulates a comparable increase in serum GH concentrations in both sedentary and fit people. However sedentary people experience higher GH levels for several hours after intense activity compared to fit ones. Submaximal exercise provokes a greater GH response in sedentary people compared to fit ones, meaning that sedentary people are less fit and thus experience submaximal exercise as a more of a physical stressor than fit subjects do.

Thyroid-Stimulating Hormone

The release of TSH from the anterior pituitary lobe can increase during exercise, but it does not appear to do so consistently. The section titled Thyroid Hormones describes thyroid gland secretions during exercise.

Posterior Pituitary Hormones

The posterior pituitary lobe stores and secretes ADH and oxytocin, which are transported from the hypothalamus. Little information is available about the effects of exercise on oxytocin. However evidence supports the idea that exercise is a potent stimulus for ADH secretion.

During periods of heavy sweating and intense exercise, ADH works to minimise the extent of water loss from the kidneys, thereby decreasing the risk of severe dehydration. This response helps the body conserve fluids, especially during exercise in the heat, when a person is most at risk for dehydration. By increasing the water permeability of the kidneys' collecting ducts, ADH facilitates the conservation of water, allowing less water to be excreted in the urine.

With intense muscular work and heavy perspiration, the electrolytes become more concentrated in the blood plasma, which increases the plasma *osmolality* (the ionic concentration of dissolved substances, such as electrolytes, in the plasma). Additionally, sweating causes water to be drawn out of the blood, resulting in a lower plasma volume. The hypothalamus can sense increased plasma osmolality and lowered plasma volume, and responds by stimulating the posterior pituitary lobe to secrete ADH (see figure 10.6). In contrast, ADH secretion is minimised when fluid intake increases and the blood volume expands, resulting in more dilute urine.

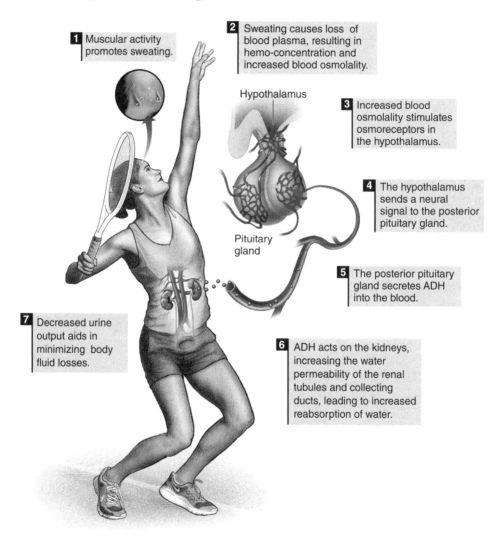

1 Muscular activity promotes sweating.

2 Sweating causes loss of blood plasma, resulting in hemo-concentration and increased blood osmolality.

Hypothalamus

3 Increased blood osmolality stimulates osmoreceptors in the hypothalamus.

4 The hypothalamus sends a neural signal to the posterior pituitary gland.

Pituitary gland

5 The posterior pituitary gland secretes ADH into the blood.

7 Decreased urine output aids in minimizing body fluid losses.

6 ADH acts on the kidneys, increasing the water permeability of the renal tubules and collecting ducts, leading to increased reabsorption of water.

Figure 10.6 Antidiuretic hormone's influence on the conservation of body water during exercise.

Reprinted, by permission, from W.L. Kenney, J.W. Wilmore, and D.L. Costill, 2015, *Physiology of sport and exercise*, 6th ed. (Champaign, IL: Human Kinetics), 112.

Thyroid Hormones

The thyroid gland secretes T_3 and T_4 (general metabolic hormones) and calcitonin, which facilitates calcium metabolism. T_3 and T_4 are involved in the following important functions:

- Regulation of *basal metabolic rate*
- Protein and enzyme synthesis
- Increasing the size and number of *mitochondria* in most cells
- Rapid cellular uptake of glucose
- *Glycolysis* and gluconeogenesis
- Lipid mobilisation, increasing FFAs for use in aerobic metabolism

TSH stimulates the thyroid and controls the release of T_3 and T_4. During exercise plasma T_4 concentrations do increase, but a delay occurs between T_4 elevations and TSH concentrations, so it is unclear whether there is a direct causal relationship between these two hormones during exercise. During submaximal aerobic endurance exercise there is a sharp initial increase in T_4 concentrations, but then T_4 remains relatively constant at a lower level throughout the rest of the bout. During prolonged submaximal exercise, T_3 concentrations tend to decrease.

Adrenal Hormones

The adrenal gland is actually two distinct glands located atop each kidney—the adrenal medulla (inner portion), which secretes the catecholamines, and the adrenal cortex (outer portion), which secretes steroid hormones called *corticosteroids*. Generally corticosteroids are categorised as mineralocorticoids, glucocorticoids and gonadocorticoids.

Catecholamines

Epinephrine and norepinephrine (collectively called the *catecholamines*) secreted by the adrenal medulla are hormones of the sympathetic nervous system. They exert widespread effects on the organ systems that are critical for exercise performance. This readying process is often referred to as the *fight-or-flight response*, and it consists of preparing the body for strenuous physical activity in the face of an emergency or stressful situation.

Epinephrine is the primary hormone released by the adrenal medulla. Under the influence of epinephrine (and to a lesser extent, norepinephrine), the following responses occur:

- The strength of cardiac contraction increases, resulting in increased cardiac output.
- Generalised vasoconstriction in non-exercising muscles acts to increase total peripheral resistance. Combined, these effects cause an increase in SBP, thus ensuring an appropriate driving pressure to force blood to the organs most vital for physical exertion.
- Vasodilation of heart and active skeletal-muscle blood vessels occurs. Skeletal muscle vasodilation is then maintained throughout the course of the exercise session through auto-regulation, which is affected by the by-products created during muscle metabolism.
- Epinephrine (but not norepinephrine) dilates the respiratory passages to aid in moving air into and out of the lungs, and reduces digestive activity and bladder emptying during exercise.
- Blood glucose concentration is also influenced by the release of epinephrine.
    - In general epinephrine stimulates the mobilisation of stored carbohydrate and fat for the purpose of making them available as energy to fuel muscular work.
    - Specifically epinephrine stimulates the production (gluconeogenesis) and release (*glycogenolysis*) of liver glycogen. It also stimulates glycogenolysis in skeletal muscles.
    - Epinephrine also increases blood fatty-acid levels by promoting *lipolysis* (the breakdown of triglycerides in adipose tissue to FFAs for use as fuel).
- Lastly epinephrine affects the central nervous system by promoting a state of arousal and increased alertness to permit quick thinking to help cope with the impending stressor (or exercise activity).

During physical exertion, blood levels of epinephrine and norepinephrine increase linearly with the duration of exercise. Norepinephrine increases noticeably until exercise intensity approaches 50 percent of $\dot{V}O_2max$, whereas epinephrine levels remain unchanged until exercise intensity exceeds about 60 percent of $\dot{V}O_2max$. These fast-acting hormones function to mobilise glucose and free fatty acids to maintain blood glucose concentration.

Cortisol

Glucocorticoids facilitate the control of consistent plasma glucose concentrations and mobilisation of fatty acids. Cortisol (also called hydrocortisone) is the major glucocorticoid released from the adrenal cortex, and accounts for approximately 95 percent of all glucocorticoid presence in the body. Cortisol contributes to FFA mobilisation from adipose tissue, glucose synthesis in the liver (i.e., gluconeogenesis) and a decrease in the rate of glucose utilisation by the cells. Its effect is slow, however, allowing other fast-acting hormones, such as epinephrine and glucagon, to primarily deal with glucose and FFA mobilisation. Besides glucose control, cortisol also acts to stimulate protein breakdown to release amino acids for use in repair and energy production, works as an anti-inflammatory agent, depresses immune reactions and works synergistically with epinephrine to increase vasoconstriction.

Cortisol production increases with exercise intensity and with increasing levels of stress placed on the body's physiological systems. During an acute bout of cardiorespiratory exercise, plasma cortisol concentration peaks after 30 to 45 minutes and then decreases to close-to-normal levels. Extremely high cortisol levels occur after long-duration events such as a marathon. This postexercise elevation suggests that cortisol plays a role in tissue recovery and repair. However, prolonged elevations in blood cortisol levels have been linked with excessive protein breakdown, tissue wasting, negative nitrogen balance and abdominal obesity. People who follow very low-carbohydrate, low-calorie weight-loss diets often experience ketosis (i.e., dangerously excessive keto-acid concentrations in the extracellular fluid), which is amplified by elevated cortisol secretion.

Aldosterone

Mineralocorticoids play an important role in regulating extracellular electrolyte balance. Aldosterone is the major mineralocorticoid released from the adrenal cortex, and accounts for most (at least 95 percent) of all mineralocorticoid activity. Aldosterone affects electrolyte balance by promoting the reabsorption of sodium in the kidneys, which results in overall retention of bodily sodium. Water follows sodium such that an increase in sodium also results in fluid retention within the body and an increase in blood pressure. Additionally, sodium retention causes potassium excretion, which means that aldosterone also affects potassium balance. Thus the following factors stimulate aldosterone release:

- Decreased plasma sodium
- Decreased blood volume
- Decreased blood pressure
- Increased plasma concentration

Together with ADH, aldosterone works to conserve the body's fluid content, which helps to minimise plasma volume loss, maintain blood pressure and prevent dehydration. The effects of ADH and aldosterone are at work during exercise. These effects persist for up to 48 hours after a bout of exercise, leading to a reduction in urine production and, consequently, a decreased risk for dehydration.

Pancreatic Hormones

The pancreas is the endocrine gland responsible for the majority of hormonal actions relating to plasma glucose regulation. The pancreas secretes insulin and glucagon, which work in opposition to control the amount of glucose circulating in the blood.

Insulin

Insulin is directly involved in the uptake of glucose into tissue. Essentially insulin exerts a hypoglycaemic effect by reducing blood glucose levels and promoting the uptake of glucose, fats and amino acids into cells for storage. During physical activity, however, the body needs to mobilise stored forms of fuel to use for energy. Therefore the effects of insulin would generally be considered counterproductive. Activation of the sympathetic system during exercise suppresses insulin release from the pancreas. Glucose uptake by skeletal muscle can increase 7 to 20 times over the values observed at rest. Muscle tissue can take up higher levels of glucose at a faster rate, even when insulin levels are decreasing, partly due to an increase in muscle's sensitivity to insulin even after an acute bout of exercise training. As a result, less insulin is needed to bring about the same effect on glucose uptake into muscle tissue.

Glucagon

Another hormone released by the pancreas, glucagon, has the opposite effect of insulin on blood glucose concentrations. Glucagon stimulates an almost instantaneous release of glucose from the liver, and is part of a negative feedback loop in which low blood glucose levels stimulate its release. In other words, one of glucagon's primary roles is to facilitate an increase in blood glucose concentration. Glucagon primarily contributes to blood glucose control as exercise progresses and glycogen stores deplete. This typically happens later, rather than earlier, in an exercise bout. Working together, insulin and glucagon favour the maintenance of blood glucose levels at a time when the muscle is using blood glucose at a high rate.

Gonadal Hormones

Testosterone produced by the testes and oestrogen and progesterone produced by the ovaries are the major gonadal hormones. In males testosterone increases during a bout of exercise; in females oestrogen and progesterone levels are elevated with exercise. Although the role of oestrogen and progesterone in exercise metabolism is unclear, testosterone has a direct effect on muscle tissue synthesis. Because most of testosterone's exercise-related effects are observed after a period of chronic training, more details about testosterone and exercise are presented in the following section.

Hormonal Adaptations to Chronic Exercise Training

In general, the hormonal response to a given exercise load declines with regular aerobic endurance training. This increased efficiency may result from improved target tissue sensitivity or responsiveness to a given amount of hormone. A selection of hormones and their general responses to aerobic endurance exercise is listed below. Resistance training also brings about hormonal response alterations, particularly with testosterone and GH.

- Epinephrine and norepinephrine. Decreased secretion of epinephrine and norepinephrine at rest and at the same absolute exercise intensity after training.
- Slight deviation of cortisol during exercise.
- Increased sensitivity to insulin; normal decrease in insulin during exercise greatly reduced with training.
- Smaller increase in glucose levels during exercise at absolute and relative workloads.
- No effect on resting values of growth hormone; less dramatic rise during exercise.

Adrenal Hormones

Catecholamine (i.e., epinephrine and norepinephrine) output declines significantly during the first several weeks of submaximal aerobic endurance training. The favourable training adaptations of a lowered resting heart rate and a smaller rise in blood pressure during submaximal exercise are the most common evidence of decreased catecholamine levels. Circulating cortisol levels tend to increase slightly as a result of exercise training as the body seeks to become more efficient at preserving glucose.

Pancreatic Hormones

People who participate in regular aerobic endurance exercise maintain blood levels of insulin and glucagon during exercise that are closer to resting values. This is important because the trained state requires less insulin at any specific point from rest through submaximal-intensity exercise. In addition the combination of resistance exercise and aerobic training improves the insulin sensitivity of active muscles more than aerobic training alone. Thus people with blood glucose regulation problems (i.e., those with metabolic syndrome or diabetes) stand to benefit from both modes of exercise training.

Growth Hormone

People who regularly do aerobic endurance exercise show less rise in circulating blood growth hormone levels at a given exercise intensity than their untrained counterparts. This can be attributed to the reduction in physiological stress that occurs as a result of the exercise stimulus as training progresses and fitness improves. In contrast resistance training augments growth hormone release (via increases in testosterone) and interacts with nervous system function to increase muscle force production, especially in men.

Testosterone

In addition to growth hormone, testosterone is a primary hormone that affects resistance-training adaptations. Heavy resistance exercise (i.e., 85 to 95 percent of *one-repetition maximum* [*1RM*]), or moderate- to high-volume training with multiple sets or exercises with less than 1-minute rest intervals, along with training larger muscle groups, leads to an increase in testosterone release (Kraemer, W.J. (1988). Following long-term resistance training in men, resting testosterone levels increase, which is associated with strength improvement over time.

Conclusion

Almost all aspects of human function are influenced by the endocrine system. Hormones regulate growth, metabolism, sexual development and function, and responses to stress (including the body's responses to acute exercise and chronic physical training). Hormones generally fit into one of two categories: steroid hormones and non-steroid hormones. The chemical make-up of hormones determines how they interact with target sites throughout the body. When hormones are released into the bloodstream, they are carried to a specific organ or tissue containing target cells where they can perform their intended functions. The endocrine system uses a negative feedback system to regulate many of the hormonal actions in the body. The endocrine system plays a significant role in controlling physiological functions during acute exercise as well as in the adaptations that occur as a result of chronic exercise.

Lifestyle
Assessment ⇒⇒⇒⇒⇒

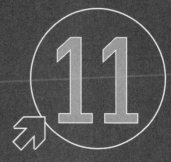

Health and Fitness Assessment

Nuno Pimenta

Samantha Jones

Ben Jones

Health and fitness assessment is foundational in the professional tasks demanded from any personal trainer. Only by assessing a client's health and fitness status can a personal trainer fully deliver the personal feature of the job. Overall the health and fitness assessment will help personal trainers design safe, highly tuned and individualised exercise programmes, better define realistic exercise goals, accurately monitor a client's progression and readjust the initial exercise program. This chapter provides current information and guidelines on how to assess clients' health status and overall fitness in a personal training setting.

Defining Health and Fitness

Health and fitness are two basic concepts that define a whole professional and research field. Both concepts have been comprehensively defined in the literature. Though they are rather broad concepts, they should be used accurately and meaningfully. The term *health*, as adopted in the World Health Organization (WHO) Constitution since the 1946 New York conference, refers to 'a state of complete physical, mental and social well-being and not merely the absence of disease or infirmity' (WHO 2009, p. 1).

Fitness (originally called *physical fitness*) refers to 'a set of attributes that people have or achieve' related to the 'ability to carry out daily tasks with vigor and alertness, without undue fatigue and with ample energy to enjoy leisure-time pursuits and to meet unforeseen emergencies' (Caspersen et al. 1985, p. 128). This definition was subsequently endorsed by the United States Surgeon General (CDC 1996), and it has been generally accepted in the field of health and fitness (Thompson 2013).

The initial definition by Caspersen and colleagues (1985) included a distinction between health-related fitness and skill-related fitness. *Health-related fitness* and its components have been proposed to be highly related to and important for public health. Despite the fact that *skill-related fitness* components such as muscle power are increasingly thought to have implications for public health, this chapter focuses mainly on health-related fitness, sometimes referred to just as *fitness*, and on its components. Health-related fitness includes five components: body composition, cardiorespiratory endurance (often called cardiorespiratory fitness), muscular endurance, muscular strength and flexibility. All of the health-related fitness components are related to the ability to perform physical activity, but these fitness components are also highly related to health outcomes. For more details about health- and skill-related fitness, see chapter 6 of *EuropeActive's Foundations for Exercise Professionals* (Iglesias-Soler and Chapman 2015).

Preliminary Health Assessment

Before conducting any exercise-related assessments the personal trainer must gather insightful knowledge about the client's health status and exercise-related risk of health complications. This knowledge is absolutely necessary for assuring exercise safety and assisting clients to meet their goals in an effective and safe manner.

EuropeActive has published simple and sound guidelines for health screening and risk assessment (Santos-Rocha and Pimenta 2015) following standardised approaches (CSEP 2013; Greenland et al. 2010; ACSM 2013). Even though more extensive and deeper approaches may be considered, EuropeActive recommends that readers consult chapter 15 of *EuropeActive's Foundations for Exercise Professionals* (Santos-Rocha and Pimenta 2015), which describes these components in detail, including various forms and standards:

- Physical Activity Readiness Questionnaire (PAR-Q)
- Health appraisal and risk assessment
- Exercise-related cardiac risk classification

- EACPR's model for cardiovascular evaluation
- ACSM's model for risk classification

Fitness Assessments

After the personal trainer has conducted a preliminary health assessment and cleared clients to engage in or increase exercise participation, clients are now ready for fitness assessment. The tests that constitute an overall fitness assessment should not be fixed, but should instead be individualised and fine-tuned for each client. Table 11.1 shows a simple but robust assessment model based on a three-level approach that simultaneously standardises and individualises each client's assessment protocol. In simple terms the personal trainer will choose the intensity (level 1, 2 or 3) of the approach that is necessary for each health related fitness component for each client. For example clients who are highly focused on body composition may have their body composition assessed on level 3, muscle strength and cardiorespiratory fitness assessed on level 2 and muscle endurance and flexibility on level 1. On the other hand a client highly focused on overall well-being could have all health-related fitness components assessed on level 1. A different client, highly focused on

Table 11.1 Health-Related Fitness Component Assessment Model

Health-related fitness component	Level 1	Level 2	Level 3
Body composition	BMI + WC + HC + bioimpedance	Level 1 + full-body anthropometric profile	Level 2 + DXA
Cardiorespiratory fitness	Non-exercise $\dot{V}O_2$ estimation	Submaximal field test or laboratory (or some health clubs) test	Laboratory (or some health clubs) maximal tests
Muscle endurance	No assessment	Push-up test Curl-up test Sit-up test Plank hold	Same as level 2
Muscle strength	No assessment	1RM prediction methods	1RM evaluation (directly measured)
Flexibility	Sit-and-reach test	Level 1 + back-scratch test; shoulder elevation test	Level 2 + goniometry

BMI = body mass index; WC = waist circumference; HC = hip circumference; DXA = dual-energy X-ray absorptiometry; 1RM = one-repetition maximum.

performance, should have higher precision in fitness assessment, and therefore could be assessed on level 3 in all components. The idea is that a fitness assessment can and should be individualised and that the instruments selected should be adjusted to be at least age, sex and race specific.

The remainder of this chapter presents procedures and specificities regarding a fitness assessment. It is organised into two subsections. The first is *pre-exercise assessments*, including all assessments that should be conducted at rest. Results may be altered or disturbed if assessment is done after the client is engaged in any testing involving physical activity effort or exercise. The second is *health-related fitness component assessments*, which involve exercise testing. Before a fitness assessment, however, the personal trainer and the client should go through the informed consent process and the client should fill in and sign an informed consent form.

Informed Consent Process and Form

Informed consent is the process of obtaining the client's signature to confirm that they have read and received a satisfactory explanation of the benefits, limitations and risks of engaging in the services being offered. Clients must be aware that their consent needs to be given freely and that they have the right to withdraw this consent and stop an exercise test or programme or terminate any other service at any time. Informed consent must be obtained from a client prior to beginning any process in a professional capacity. This includes when a personal trainer collects a client's personal information, conducts fitness assessments, provides lifestyle advice, designs an exercise programme or instructs exercise.

The normal method for obtaining informed consent is to provide the client with a form and to explain its content, giving the client the opportunity to ask questions prior to signing the form. This signature represents their consent for the collection of personal information and participation in the services offered.

An informed consent form should contain the following information:

- Client personal details (full name, date of birth, contact details)
- Details of the proposed services (e.g., a detailed description of fitness testing procedures)
- Client's right to choose to terminate or withdraw from services (e.g., to choose not to be weighed) or to finish a fitness test prior to the desired end point
- Assurance of confidentiality

- Statement that participation is voluntary
- Statement that clients can ask any questions they may have prior to giving consent
- Client's signature and the date

The informed consent form is a legal document that contains personal information belonging to the client. It must therefore be treated confidentially according to the organisation's information governance policy. At a minimum this is likely to include the following:

- Not divulging the client's personal details to a third party
- Safe and secure storage of the form
- Retaining the form, along with other legal documents, for a predetermined length of time depending on national legislation and local policy

Pre-Exercise Assessments

Pre-exercise assessments include all assessments that should be conducted before exercise or exercise testing. This is mainly because exercise and the associated increase in metabolic rate, as well as all physiologic responses to exercise, may influence results, compromising data accuracy and its ability to reflect resting steady state.

Resting Blood Pressure

Blood pressure (BP) is the force that blood exerts in the inner wall of the arteries and veins; it is created by the pumping force of the heart (ACSM 2013). Arterial BP is the one usually assessed. It is measured in units of millimetres of mercury (mmHg), and varies considerably in between two heartbeats (systoles). *Systolic blood pressure* (SBP) is the maximum BP observed immediately after a systole due to the effort exerted by the cardiac muscle (ACSM 2007). *Diastolic blood pressure* (DBP) is the minimum BP observed during the diastole (relaxation of the heart) and immediately before a systole (ACSM 2007). Blood pressure optimal values are proposed to be 120 mmHg for SBP and 80 mmHg for DBP (tables 11.2 and 11.3; Chobanian et al. 2003; WHO 2003).

Hypertension (HT) is diagnosed when resting BP (either SBP or DBP) is chronically above cutoff values of 140 or 90 mmHg for SBP and DBP, respectively. Table 11.2 shows the guidelines from the World Health Organization (WHO) and the sixth report of the Joint National Committee (JNC) for the United States National Institutes of Health (NIH), which define three categories of BP under HT and three HT levels (NIH 1997; WHO 2003). The seventh report of the

Table 11.2 Blood Pressure Classification for Adults

	Blood pressure			
	SBP (mmHg)			DBP (mmHg)
Optimal	<120		and	<80
Normal	<130		and	<85
High-normal	130-139		or	85-89
Hypertension				
Level 1	140-159		or	90-99
Level 2	160-179		or	100-109
Level 3	≥180		or	≥110

SBP = systolic blood pressure; DBP = diastolic blood pressure.
According to the Sixth Joint National Committee Report (NIH 1997) and the World Health Organization (WHO 2003).

Table 11.3 Blood Pressure Classification for Adults

	Blood pressure			
	SBP (mmHg)			DBP (mmHg)
Normal	<120		and	<80
Pre-HT	120-139		or	80-89
Level 1 HT	140-59		or	90-99
Level 2 HT	≥160		or	≥100

SBP = systolic blood pressure; DBP = diastolic blood pressure; HT = hypertension.
National Institutes of Health (NIH) 1997.

JNC presents a rather simpler classification (table 11.3), including only two categories of BP under HT, emphasising the risk of hypertension, and only two HT levels (Chobanian et al. 2003).

High values of resting blood pressure may result from increased work of the heart pump, increasing both the volume of blood being pumped in each beat and the number of beats per minute (*heart rate*) and resulting in an increased *cardiac output* (amount of blood coming out of the heart per minute). This happens as a normal response to exercise. However BP may be pathologically increased at rest. This happens mainly as a result of increased stiffness in the arteries and reduced compliance of arteries in regard to blood flow, increasing the resistance offered to blood flow in systemic circulation (*total peripheral resistance*).

Hypertension has been found to be present in at least 30 percent of the population in developed countries (Costa et al. 2003; Fields et al. 2004). It is considered to be a risk factor for the development of cardiovascular diseases (CVD), with the risk of developing CVD increasing twofold if there are increases of 20 mmHg (SBP) or 10 mmHg (DBP) within an overall BP range of 115/75 mmHg to 185/110 mmHg (Chobanian et al. 2003).

Resting blood pressure is an important component of resting, or pre-exercise, assessments. The result of BP assessment can be used in risk classification models, and is also important for determining exercise prescription adjustments and setting intervention goals according to the client's specificity and needs. The direct assessment of BP is highly invasive, involving the intra-arterial placement of a pressure gauge, and cannot be conducted by the personal trainer. BP is routinely assessed using indirect methods.

BP can be indirectly assessed using an automated system or a manual aneroid manometer. Automated assessment of BP requires electronic BP assessment equipment, which is available in many clinical settings such as doctor offices and hospitals, as well as in gyms and health clubs. Commercial models have become rather inexpensive, allowing independent personal trainers to use them with their clients. Although automated devices are suggested to provide reasonably accurate BP measurements, they often are difficult to calibrate, which may compromise readings over time (ACSM 2013).

Manual assessment of BP requires a stethoscope to listen to (*auscultate*) the Korotkoff sounds (table 11.4) and a sphygmomanometer, which includes an inflation system and a manometer (mercury or aneroid) for measuring pressure. The inflation system consists of a non-distensible cuff that can be securely wrapped around the limb and an inflation bulb for manual inflation of the bladder in the cuff. The cuff of the inflating system should encase an expandable rectangular rubber bladder. The rubber bladder should be neither too big (big rubber bladders tend to underestimate BP) nor too small (small rubber bladders significantly overestimate BP). Recommendations state that the rubber bladder's width and length should be 40 and 80 percent of arm circumference, respectively (Perloff et al. 1993).

Table 11.4 The Five Phases of Korotkoff Sounds (Perloff et al. 1993)

Phases of Korotkoff sounds	Description
Phase 1	First appearance of clear, repetitive tapping sounds. This coincides approximately with the reappearance of palpable pulse.
Phase 2	Sounds are softer and longer with the quality of an intermittent murmur.
Phase 3	Sounds again become crisper and louder.
Phase 4	Sounds are muffled, less distinct and softer.
Phase 5	Sounds disappear completely.

The tubing of the inflation system connects both the manometer and the inflation bulb to the bladder.

The assessment of BP should follow an accurate protocol so that results obtained from the measurement are reliable. Though a comprehensive BP measurement protocol is fully described elsewhere (Perloff et al. 1993), the sidebar "Protocol for Blood Pressure Measurement" presents a summary of the basic procedures for a proper measurement.

Resting Heart Rate

Resting heart rate (HRrest) is the number of systoles that occur in a specific time frame. Usually HRrest is expressed in beats (systoles) per minute. Heart rate (HR) is highly controlled by the autonomic nervous system (ANS) in response to physiological challenges such as orthostasis, thermic regulation or exercise and subsequent recovery (Haqq et al. 2012; Riganello et al. 2012).

The parasympathetic nervous system (PNS) branch of the ANS exerts an inhibitory effect through the vagal nerve, reducing HR and ventricular contractility so that the heart is not exposed to excessive

⇒⇒⇒ Protocol for Blood Pressure Measurement (Chobanian et al. 2003; Perloff et al. 1993).

Basic aspects of indirect measurement of BP:
- Conducted through auscultation
- Has a standard estimation error of about 10%, when compared with direct measurement
- Carried out with properly calibrated equipment
- SBP is defined as the point at which the first of several Korotkoff sounds is heard (phase 1)
- DBP is defined as the point immediately before Korotkoff sounds disappear completely (phase 5)
- Feedback regarding BP assessment, as well as BP goals, should be provided to all clients, preferably both verbal and written.

Preliminary procedures for the measurement of BP:
- Clients should be provided with information about the assessment as part of the informed consent form.
- Client should rest for at least 5 minutes, seated in a chair, before the measurement of BP.
- For measurement client should be seated, with back supported, feet flat on the floor and arm supported at heart level.

Procedures for manual indirect measurement of BP:
- The result of BP measurement should be the average of at least two measurements.

unnecessary work (Seals 2006). At rest PNS is dominant in the control of cardiac function, which causes the sinoatrial node to decrease HR (Widmaier et al. 2011). In the complete absence of any influence, neither hormonal nor neural, the sinoatrial node pace is about 100 beats per minute; however most people have lower heart rates at rest due to PNS action (Widmaier et al. 2011).

At the onset of exercise, many times even before the start of actual exercise, HR increases in response to decreases in PNS activity to the vagal nerve, affecting the sinoatrial node and the ventricular muscle of the heart, which then reduce the tonic suppressive effect of the vagal cardiac stimulation on HR and ventricular contractility (Seals 2006). This highlights the volatility of HRrest, meaning that simply thinking about exercising may be enough to increase HR.

Heart rate is highly changeable; therefore the use of a comprehensive protocol for its assessment is vital for obtaining accurate readings. By definition true HRrest should be measured in the morning right after waking up (Wilmore and Costill 2004). Since this is somewhat unrealistic for personal trainers, they have two options: Clients may self-assess their HRrest in the morning right

- Expose the client's arm up to the shoulder, making sure that the arm is not being tightened by clothing.
- Position the arm in a supine position with the palm of the hand facing up.
- Place the cuff around the upper right arm with the rubber bladder covering the radial artery. It should not be too tight.
- Place the head of the stethoscope over the client's radial artery, slightly in the inside of the arm just above the anterior curve of the elbow.
- Place the stethoscope ear tips in your ears and close the valve of the inflation bulb by rotating it clockwise.
- Inflate the cuff rapidly by pressing successively the inflation bulb to just 20 to 30 mmHg above estimated SBP (based on previous measurements).
- When previous BP of the client is not known, inflate the cuff to at least 200 mmHg.
- Slowly release the pressure of the cuff at a rate of 2 to 3 mmHg/sec, listening for Korotkoff sounds.
- When the first Korotkoff sound is heard, immediately register the value of SBP.
- Continue to release pressure until you hear the last Korotkoff sound (DBP).
- Deflate the cuff rapidly when the Korotkoff sounds disappear completely.
- Do not inflate the cuff again immediately if the reading has failed.
- If a BP reading fails, completely empty the cuff and let the client rest for 2 to 3 minutes before measuring BP again.

BP = blood pressure; SBP = systolic blood pressure; DBP = diastolic blood pressure.

after waking up, following instructed guidelines, or the personal trainer may control the measurement protocol and apply it with the client at another point in the day. To assure higher accuracy HRrest should be assessed in the morning, preferably after sleeping through the night (in a fasting state).

Several techniques for measuring HR can be used to assess HRrest: palpation of a standardised anatomical site (radial artery or carotid artery), auscultation of the heart using a stethoscope placed directly on the chest (care should be taken to count systole and diastole as one beat), electronic HR monitors or watches and the electrocardiogram. The use of electronic HR monitors or watches is quite simple and handy for assessing HR in all sorts of situations, including rest, exercise and recovery. Electrocardiograms are not accessible to most personal trainers, even those affiliated with health clubs; therefore this chapter does not focus on them.

Body Composition

Body composition, despite being assessed pre-exercise, is the first health related fitness component to be assessed both because it does not influence subsequent assessments and because it may be influenced by prior exercise involved assessments (e.g. any sweating may dramatically influence weight and bio-impedance results, reducing weight and overestimating body fat; and strength assessments may influence anthropometrics, particularly increasing the limb's circumferences). For this reason, body composition is mentioned here in the pre-exercise assessments rather than in the subsections relative to fitness components assessment, even though body composition is a recognized health related fitness component.

The study of body composition (BC) is strongly associated with (and sometimes confused with) the study of obesity. However the study of BC includes body components far beyond fat mass alone. Body composition is considered a component of health-related fitness, and it has been proven to have physical, morphological and particularly important health implications (CDC 1996).

The study of BC is a fascinating branch of the biological sciences. Over the years a wide variation has been observed in the terminology and methodology used for its assessment. The terminology and the five-level model suggested by Wang and colleagues (figure 11.1) was a milestone in the field of BC assessment. They are still fairly commonly used, despite more recent technological advances. In the five-level model, it is assumed that each component within each level is mutually exclusive, and that the sum of all the components in the same level is equivalent to whole body mass (Wang et al. 1992). The atomic level includes 11 major components, including oxygen,

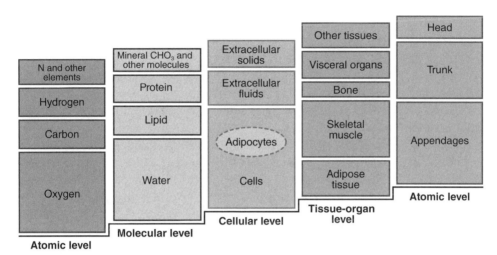

Figure 11.1   The five-level model in body composition suggested by Wang and colleagues. N = nitrogen; CHO = carbohydrates.

Adapted, by permission, from W. Shen, M. St-Onge, Z. Wang, and S. Heymsfield, 2005, Study of body composition: An overview. In *Human Body Composition,* 2nd ed., edited by S. Heymsfield, T.G. Lohman, Z. Wang, and S. Going. (Champaign, IL: Human Kinetics), 4.

hydrogen, carbon and nitrogen, which together account for more than 96 percent of whole body mass (Shen et al. 2005). These atoms constitute molecules including water, lipids, carbohydrate, protein, bone minerals and soft-tissue minerals, which are the six major components at the molecular level (Shen et al. 2005). The molecular level is probably one of the most widely considered levels in BC analysis. At the molecular level it is possible to use multicomponent models: the widely used two-compartment model (body fat [BF] + fat-free mass), which can be assessed by most methods available, or the three-compartment model (BF + bone mineral content + lean soft tissue), which can be assessed by dual-energy X-ray absorptiometry (DXA; Shen et al. 2005).

The commonly used word *fat* may be used interchangeably with BF. It refers to triglycerides, the molecular form in which lipids are stored in the body. BF can be stored in the adipose tissue and in other tissues as well. At the cellular level it is important to distinguish between adipose tissue and the widely studied BF or lipids, the latest component to be assessed at the molecular level (figure 11.2; Shen et al. 2005). Lipids include non-fat lipids (those not in the form of triglycerides), which are found both in adipose and other tissues, lipids stored within the adipose tissue in the form of triglycerides and lipids in the form of triglycerides stored in other tissues. Adipose tissue comprises BF and non-fat lipids, such as phospholipids, but includes also other components essential to the survival and function of adipose tissue cells. About 80 percent of adipose tissue is fat and the remainder 20 percent is made of water, protein and minerals (Shen et al., 2003).

The fifth level, the whole-body level, can be assessed using simple measures of weight or height, and can also be divided into regions such as the head, limbs and trunk, which can be assessed with various anthropometric techniques, such as circumference, skinfold and length.

Chapter 10 of *EuropeActive's Foundations for Exercise Professionals* (Carnero & Garcia, 2015) covers body composition assessment using both bio-electric impedance (BIA) and anthropometrics. Comprehensive descriptions of anthropometric measurements can be found elsewhere (Lohman at al., 1988; Marfell-Jones et al., 2006). We do recommend that any anthropometric measurement protocol be used consistently, as modification of the measurement protocol may result in biased unusable data. Additionally DXA may be used to assess body composition, in a three-compartment model (body fat, bone mass and lean soft tissue—which is body mass free of bone and fat), of the whole body or body regions. DXA cannot identify adipose tissue. Some attempts, however, have been made to estimate visceral adipose tissue using DXA, with promising results (Kamel et al. 2000; Park et al. 2002). Yet DXA gives precise estimates only of whole body composition (body fat, bone mass and lean soft tissue) as well as of specific regions or segments of the body, including the upper and lower limbs, the trunk or the abdominal regions and other customised regions if needed (Lohman and Chen 2005). For clarifying purposes this chapter adopts the terminology recommended

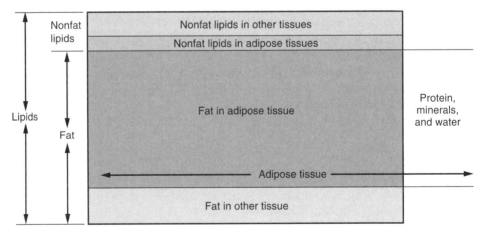

Figure 11.2 Relationships among the molecular-level components lipid and fat and the tissue-organ-level component adipose tissue.

Adapted, by permission, from W. Shen, M. St-Onge, Z. Wang, and S. Heymsfield, 2005, Study of body composition: An overview. In *Human Body Composition,* 2nd ed., edited by S. Heymsfield, T.G. Lohman, Z. Wang, and S. Going. (Champaign, IL: Human Kinetics), 12.

by Sardinha and Teixeira (2005): *whole BF* refers to the whole body, *regional BF* represents a single variable of a body region, as in total abdominal fat, and *BF distribution* refers to the measurement of one variable in relation to another so that a dichotomous fat distribution type can be identified (e.g., a contrast or a ratio), as expressed in Vague's pioneer observations on this topic (Vague 1950; 1956). Nevertheless it is recognised that the expressions *regional BF* and *BF distribution* have been commonly used interchangeably (Sardinha and Teixeira 2005).

The proposed three-level model for determining fitness assessment intensity helps personal trainers make appropriate and rapid choices when individualising the assessment of health-related fitness components, which is particularly relevant in the case of body composition. The choice for level 1, when level 2 is not needed, will save the personal trainer a lot of time, whilst the choice for level 2, when level 3 is not needed, will save the client a lot of money. On the other hand the choice for level 2 when level 1 is insufficient may make a difference for the client in achieving their goals and for the personal trainer in monitoring and identifying the client's achievements. Table 11.1 provides a succinct presentation of the three-level model as applied to body composition assessment. The minimum full body anthropometric assessment, recommended in level 2 and 3, should include, additionally to weight and height (mandatory in all levels), circumferences and skinfolds measurement of every body segment (table 11.5).

Posture and Body Alignment

Another static measurement that has become increasingly popular with personal trainers and expected by clients is the evaluation of posture. This typically involves static and dynamic tests or observations that can be recorded in a standardised way to monitor changes in the client's posture over time. Using a model of optimal posture such as a plumb line or posture grid provides a simple and objective

Table 11.5   Minimal Full Body Anthropometric Assessment Protocol, Other Than Weight, Height and BMI

Body region	Circumferences	Skinfold
Arm	Relaxed arm circumference	Biceps skinfold Triceps skinfold
Trunk	Waist circumference Hip circumference	Subscapular skinfold Suprailiac skinfold Abdominal skinfold
Thigh	Medial thigh circumference	Thigh skinfold
Calf	Calf circumference	Calf skinfold

snapshot of static body position on the occasion of the consultation. A photographic record may be made, with the client's express consent, or alternatively a posture observation form completed, noting observations such as 'a forward head position' or 'the right shoulder is 2 centimetres lower than the left'.

Static posture should be observed from the anterior, posterior and lateral aspects and the observations compared to give a holistic impression of the client, rather than being reduced to minutiae of a specific body part being out of perfect alignment. In optimal posture the structure of the body maintains an upright position with minimal muscular effort, the spine exhibits a neutral alignment, with its natural curves neither too great nor too small, and the relative length and strength of muscle groups are balanced across joints. This enables the client to maintain the optimal position with minimal muscular effort. The most common postural deviations are the exaggeration or reduction of the spine's natural curves.

In the neutral spine position the pelvis is aligned horizontally, providing a balanced foundation on which the lumbar vertebrae rest. The concave curve of the lumbar spine and the convex curve of the thoracic regions of the spine are sinusoidal and well balanced with one another, such that the cervical spine has a small concave curve and the head position is aligned with the pelvis, falling within the centre of gravity.

In the *hyperkyphotic posture*, although the pelvis may be in alignment (but not necessarily), the kyphotic curve is far greater than the lumbar lordosis, leading to the rounded shoulder appearance and forward head position, which necessitates an exaggerated cervical curvature to maintain a horizontal gaze. This posture has also been referred to as the *upper crossed syndrome* in a model that hypothesises a cause of muscle imbalance between key muscle groups of the neck and thorax (Page et al., 2010).

In the *hyperlordotic posture*, anterior pelvic tilt is normally exhibited, implicating muscle groups that cross the joints of the lumbar, pelvic and hip region in a *lower crossed syndrome*, where altered muscle length–tension relationships pull the lower spine into a hyperextended position to keep the thorax and head upright (Page et al., 2010).

Scoliosis is different from the other two postural deviations in that severe scoliosis is almost always caused by a congenital abnormality. It typically involves a rotated position of each vertebra on top of one another, as well as lateral curvature of the spine. In some cases scoliosis can develop due to simple mechanical muscle and connective tissue patterns reinforced by lifestyle traits such as preferentially carrying heavy shoulder or handbags on one side, carrying a child almost exclusively on one hip or regularly spending long periods of time in an awkward seated position that reinforces this lateral bend.

The main implications of postural deviations for health are musculoskeletal in nature. Lower back pain, neck pain and headaches are common. In terms of performance restricted ranges of motion at the shoulders, hips or of both regions increase risk of injury and reduce movement efficiency. In severe cases hyperkyphotic posture can reduce the size of the thoracic cavity, effectively reducing lung volume.

Posture is the product of habitual static body positions and movement patterns in a person's lifestyle that influence the arrangement of bone (Wolff's law) and connective tissues (Davis' law) according to the forces frequently placed on them. Because bone positions are determined by the forces within soft tissues, posture can be manipulated over time by changing the direction of these forces through consciously adopting new body positions. For example, a client could use a new ergonomic chair at work and practise exercises targeting specific muscle groups that would correct identified imbalances (e.g., a programme that involves stretching pectoral and latissimus dorsi muscles and resistance exercises for the lower trapezius, rhomboid and erector spinae groups) to counteract a habitually hyperkyphotic posture.

Selecting appropriate assessments for posture depends on the environment in which the consultation is taking place, the space and equipment available and the time allocated for this activity. In a client-centred model the time allocated to observe or assess posture depends primarily on how concerned the client is about their posture or whether they report any signs or symptoms that could be associated with a postural deficiency.

Besides observing standing posture from anterior, posterior and lateral positions to identify any noticeable imbalances, personal trainers may need to observe the client attempting commonly performed natural movements such as a body-weight squat or walking gait. These may help them identify abnormal movement patterns such as synergistic dominance, which could require correction of movement execution prior to initiating a loaded resistance training programme.

Other simple assessments of range of motion at specific joints or of the ability to maintain a neutral spine during a series of progressions of quadruped (horse stance) or supine (dead bug) exercises will also provide a useful indication of a client's threshold for maintaining appropriate postural alignment during exercise. These may then play a foundational role in the client's exercise programme, helping them develop core stability prior to initiating global loading in a resistance training programme. Whenever performing postural observations or assessments of flexibility or movement ability, the personal trainer should remind the client that these assessments are in no way intended to be diagnostic of any medical condition, nor is the programme designed to be a treatment for such. Professional boundaries require that if the personal trainer suspects a medical condition or the need for an assessment that they are not qualified or competent to perform, they must refer the client to an appropriate medical or health care professional.

Health-Related Fitness Component Assessments

A wide range of practical fitness assessments are available for measuring all components of fitness. The fitness test selected for each client will depend on the available equipment, environment of testing, goals, their current fitness level and their medical status. Personal trainers must consider all of these factors and explain the protocols to their clients in advance to help clients make an informed decision about whether to consent to participate in the test.

Examples of tests that can be used to evaluate each component of fitness are given here; note that the list is not exhaustive, and any validated test can be used according to a client's needs or goals:

- *Cardiorespiratory fitness:* submaximal and maximal multistage treadmill tests (e.g., Bruce or Balke), cycle ergometer tests (e.g., Astrand or YMCA), 1-mile (1.6 km) walk test, Cooper 1.5-mile (2.4 km) or 12-minute walk or run test, Queens College step test or others;
- *Muscular endurance:* push-up test, curl-up test, sit-up test, plank hold, farmer's walk among others;
- *Muscular strength:* one-repetition maximum (predicted or directly assessed) test in the squat, bench press, shoulder press, dead lift, leg press or machine chest press or other specific movements/exercises or muscle groups;
- *Flexibility:* visual observations, sit-and-reach test, goniometry, joint angle measurement (with smartphone or tablet application), overhead squat or others;
- *Motor fitness (skills):* single-leg balance, timed sprints (60 m, 100 m, 200 m), timed T-drill

The order of testing and rest periods between tests should be planned so that performance is not negatively influenced. The following test order for each health-related fitness component has been recommended: 1st - body composition; 2nd - cardiorespiratory fitness; 3rd – strength; 4th – flexibility (Arena, 2013). It may be necessary to conduct some measurements on separate testing occasions to avoid inaccuracies (e.g., after undergoing a cardiorespiratory assessment using maximal Bruce protocol the client's lower limbs may have reduced glycogen levels which reduces the capacity of exerting high levels of muscle strength and therefore influences subsequent test results). Also, to ensure that results are as meaningful as possible, on the day prior to and the day of their assessment session, clients should comply with the following:

- Avoid strenuous activity
- Not consume any alcohol
- Reschedule the assessment if they are feeling ill or have an injury
- Maintain hydration levels
- Avoid eating a large meal for at least 2 hours before the assessment
- Not eat anything for 30 minutes before the assessment
- Wear comfortable clothing and footwear that are suitable for activity
- Have a good night of sleep (e.g., 8 hours) the night before

Cardiorespiratory Fitness

The assessment of cardiorespiratory fitness (CRF) is an important part of any fitness assessment. Cardiorespiratory fitness assessment is meant to evaluate individual maximal oxygen consumption ($\dot{V}O_2$max) of a client, which is considered a key feature for the health aspect of health-related fitness and highly important for exercise prescription.

Multiple ways of characterising and classifying CRF assessment protocols exist. Field testing protocols may be applied in a wider number of settings, whilst laboratory protocols are confined to more controlled settings such as research labs and some health club facilities. Exercise protocols may also be categorised as maximal or submaximal. Maximal protocols are cardiorespiratory assessment protocols that imply that clients reach their individual maximum, whilst submaximal protocols use exercise HR during submaximal exercise to estimate individual maximal oxygen consumption.

The health-related fitness component assessment model described in table 11.1 is broadened in table 11.6 to help personal trainers make decisions about which CRF assessment to use with clients.

Non-exercise Tests Non-exercise tests, or estimation equations, are interesting alternatives when an exercise test is not intended or required. These tests usually require only resting assessments including a short query. A very interesting proposal has been validated,

Table 11.6 Three Levels of Assessment for Cardiorespiratory Fitness

Levels of assessment	Target client	Assessment procedures
Level 1	Clients concerned only with overall well-being; not concerned at all with performance	Non-exercise $\dot{V}O_2$max assessment
Level 2	Clients concerned with health and somewhat concerned with fitness, but not highly focused on performance	Field tests: 1-mile (1.6 km) walk test Cooper 1.5-mile (2.4 km) or 12-minute walk or run test Queens College step test Submaximal laboratory (or some health clubs) tests: YMCA cycle ergometer test Bruce submaximal treadmill test
Level 3	High-risk clients (in this case, any assessment must be conducted in the presence of a medical doctor), healthy clients highly focused on performance and high-performance athletes	Maximal laboratory (or some health clubs) tests: Bruce or Balke maximal treadmill test (with or without EKG and gas analysis)

including data from NASA and others, and is quite simple for the estimation of $\dot{V}O_2$max without exercise (Jurca et al. 2005). This method uses information of subjectively reported physical activity level, or the so called physical activity score (see table 11.7), along with the client's age, sex, body mass index and resting heart rate, to calculate the client's $\dot{V}O_2$max in MET. All of the mentioned data should then be included in the following formula, to find the client's $\dot{V}O_2$max in MET (Jurca et al. 2005):

$$\dot{V}O_2\text{max (MET)} = \text{sex (1 or 0)} \times 2.77 - \text{age (years)}$$
$$\times\ 0.1 - \text{BMI (kg/m}^2) \times 0.17 - \text{HRrest (bpm)} \times 0.03 + \text{PAS} + 18.07$$

For sex, enter 1 or 0 if the client is a man or a woman, respectively; for age, enter client's age in full years; BMI stands for body mass index calculated as the client's weight in kg divided by the client's squared height in meters (BMI = Weight [kg]/Height [m2]. HRrest stands for resting heart rate and is expressed in beats per minute; PAS stands for physical activity score assessed using table 11.7.

In table 11.7, the client should select the physical activity level that best describes his or her usual pattern of daily physical activ-

Table 11.7   Physical Activity Score

Description of the physical activity level	Score
Level 1 – Inactive or little activity other than usual daily activities	0.00
Level 2 – Regularly (≥5days/week) participate in physical activities requiring low levels of exertion that results in slight increasing in breathing and heart rate for at least 10 minutes at a time.	0.32
Level 3 – Participate in aerobic exercises such as brisk walking, jogging or running, cycling, swimming or vigorous sports at a comfortable pace or other activities requiring similar levels of exertion for at least 20 to 60 minutes/week.	1.06
Level 4 – Participate in aerobic exercises such as brisk walking, jogging or running, cycling, swimming or vigorous sports at a comfortable pace or other activities requiring similar levels of exertion for at least 1 to 3 hours/week.	1.76
Level 5 – Participate in aerobic exercises such as brisk walking, jogging or running, cycling, swimming or vigorous sports at a comfortable pace or other activities requiring similar levels of exertion for at least over 3 hours/week.	3.03

Adapted from Jurca et al. 2005.

ities, including activities related with household and family care, commuting, occupation, exercise and wellness as well as leisure or recreational activities. The corresponding score should be used in the estimation equation to estimate the client's $\dot{V}O_2$max in MET.

This method has a standard estimation error of about 1.5 MET, which is comparable to a lot of exercise tests available. Furthermore this is a simple approach that requires very little resources, is extremely inexpensive and allows any personal trainer to always have some information about every client's cardiorespiratory fitness. Yet exercise tests may be preferable when higher accuracy is demanded (a good selection of exercise protocols must be taken into account for this) and when the client puts a higher importance in cardiorespiratory and health-related goals.

Field Tests   Field tests are very handy for personal trainers. These tests usually require less availability of expensive pieces of equipment. They also have a wide versatility in assessment settings, meaning that CRF assessment can be conducted, for example, at the client's house with minimal resources. This can make CRF assessment the most practical and inexpensive approach. A considerable amount of validated field tests exist for the assessment of CRF.

In addition to the 12-minute Cooper test covered in chapter 19 of *EuropeActive's Foundations for Exercise Professionals* (Moody and Stevens 2015), two additional protocols can be used to assess CRF.

One-Mile (1.6 km) Walk Test

The field tests that involve locomotion require clients to cover the greatest distance in a certain amount of time or to cover a fixed distance in the least amount of time by way of walking, running or a client-determined mixture of the two. In the one-mile walk test, also called the Rockport walking test, clients are asked to walk as fast as they can to cover a full mile over-ground (Weiglein et al. 2011; Kline et al. 1987). It has been suggested that a running test could be well suited for fitter clients; however research has shown the 1-mile (1.6 km) walk test to be a valid alternative to the 1.5-mile (2.4 km) run test in assessing CRF (Weiglein et al. 2011). A standard estimation error of about 5.0 ml/kg/min has been reported for the predictive equation (Kline et al.1987).

The protocol for the 1-mile walk test developed by Kline and colleagues (1987) is simple. A client completes a full mile over-ground—by fast walking only—with the goal to complete it in the shortest amount of time. Cardiorespiratory fitness can then be assessed using the following formula:

For clients 18 to 69 years old (Weiglein et al. 2011; Kline et al. 1987):

$$\dot{V}O_2\max \text{ (ml/kg/min)} = 132.853 - 0.1692 \times \text{weight (kg)} - 0.3877 \times \text{age (years)} \\ + 6.315 \times \text{sex (0 or 1)} - 3.2649 \times \text{time (min)} - 0.1565 \times \text{HR}$$

For sex, enter 1 or 0 if the client is a man or a woman, respectively; for weight, enter client's weight, as assessed before the test; for age, enter client's age in full years; for time, enter the full time the client took to complete the full mile walk; for HR, enter the heart rate at the immediate end of the test.

The over-ground one-mile walk test has also been found feasible to be performed using a treadmill, however its usage should be selective as it was reported to underestimate high peak $\dot{V}O_2$ (Widrick et al. 1992).

Queens College Step Test

An alternative to a running or walking field test is a step test, which estimates CRF based on how quickly a client's exercise HR recovers back to HRrest immediately after a timed bench-stepping session. The faster that a client's HR returns to a resting value, the greater the client's CRF (McArdle et al. 1972).

Protocol

- Find a bench, box or step that is 41.3 centimetres (16.25 in.) high.
- Allow the client to warm up.
- Set the metronome to 88 beats per minute (women) or 96 beats per minute (men).
- Start a stopwatch or timer and direct the client to begin stepping by touching a foot (to the bench or the floor) with each beep of the metronome in an up-up-down-down cadence.
- Have the client continue stepping for 3 minutes (to reduce fatigue, the client can switch the lead leg at least once during the test).
- After 3 minutes, tell the client to stop and sit on the bench.
- Within 5 seconds of stopping the exercise, take the client's recovery HR for 15 seconds.
- Calculate the predicted $\dot{V}O_2max$ using the correct sex-specific equation:

$$\text{Men: } \dot{V}O_2max \text{ (ml/kg/min)} = 111.33 - (.42 \times \text{recovery HR})$$
$$\text{Women: } \dot{V}O_2max \text{ (ml/kg/min)} = 65.81 - (.1847 \times \text{recovery HR})$$

Advantages

- Minimal equipment needed
- Easy to administer
- Can be conducted in nearly any location

Disadvantages

- Special equipment required
- Requires an administrator

Laboratory Tests   Laboratory tests (which can also be performed in some health clubs) are often more standardised and accurate, and may be preferable for more demanding clients. These tests usually require expensive pieces of equipment (e.g., treadmill, cycle ergometers, gas-analysis system), and therefore are available in research or health-related facilities. When access to the needed equipment is available, laboratory tests are a good option for CRF assessment. A large range of maximal and submaximal CRF testing protocols can be performed in a laboratory or some health club settings. Specific test protocols have been consistently endorsed, including the YMCA submaximal test in the cycle ergometer (Beekley et al. 2004) as well as the submaximal and the maximal Bruce tests in the treadmill (Arena 2013; Bruce 1971). Personal trainers are encouraged to consult professional resources (e.g., www.brianmac.co.uk/eval.htm) for comprehensive directions, data recording sheets and nomograms, as well as multiple comprehensive guidelines elsewhere (ACSM 2013; CSEP 2013).

Muscular Endurance

Muscular endurance tests evaluate the involved muscles' ability to repeatedly contract and relax over an extended time period. A client's level of muscular endurance is specific to the part of the body and the muscles recruited to perform the test. For example the push-up test assesses the muscles of the chest (pectoralis major), front of the shoulders (anterior deltoids) and back of the upper arm (triceps), and the sit-up test assesses the muscles of the abdomen (rectus abdominis). A good score in one test does not automatically equate to a good score in the second test (although there is a sound correlation between both tests). Table 11.8 describes three levels of assessment for muscular endurance and expands on the overall health-related fitness component assessment model provided in table 11.1.

In addition to the sit-up test covered in chapter 19 of *EuropeActive's Foundations for Exercise Professionals* (Moody and Stevens 2015), an additional protocol can be used to assess a client's muscular endurance.

Table 11.8   Three Levels of Assessment for Muscular Endurance

Levels of assessment	Target client	Assessment procedures
Level 1	Clients concerned only with overall well-being and not concerned at all with performance	No assessment needed (but that does not mean that assessment is inappropriate)
Level 2	Clients somewhat concerned with performance regarding daily tasks that require strength for long periods of time	Push-up test Curl-up test Sit-up test Plank hold
Level 3	Clients highly focused in tasks involving long strength efforts or muscle endurance; high-performance athletes	The same as level 2 Additional tests may be included or developed for assessing specific sport-related tasks

Push-Up Test

Protocol

- Allow the client to warm up.
- Have the client get into the standard push-up position with the hands shoulder-width apart, elbows fully extended, and the head, shoulders, hips, knees and ankles in a straight line (figure 11.3a).
- Start a stopwatch or timer and direct the client to lower the body to the floor whilst maintaining the straight body position.

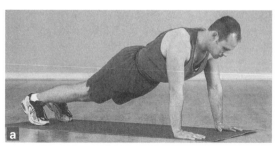

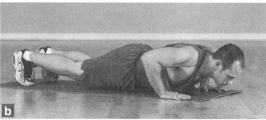

Figure 11.3 Push-up test.

- The client should continue lowering the body until the chest contacts the floor (figure 11.3b), then push back up to the starting position until the elbows are fully extended.
- Have the client continue until they cannot touch their chest to the floor in the lowest position or fully extend the elbows in the highest position.

Advantages

- Takes only a few minutes to complete
- Easy to set up and administer
- No specific equipment needed
- Can be conducted in nearly any location

Disadvantages

- Requires an administrator to monitor technique and full range of motion

For weak clients, the test assesses muscular strength rather than muscular endurance if only a minimal number of repetitions can be performed.

Muscular Strength

Muscular strength tests determine the maximum force that a client can exert in a certain movement or exercise. Like muscular endurance a client's maximum strength is specific to the muscles used to perform the test. True maximal tests require the client to lift the most weight possible in a given movement for only one repetition (1RM). This intensity level is not appropriate for all exercises or for all clients. Instead 1RM testing should be performed only with multijoint, large muscle group exercises (e.g., squat, bench press, shoulder press, dead lift, leg press or machine chest press) and for clients who are at least somewhat resistance trained and can perform the exercise properly (Baechle and Earle 2008). Refer to chapter 19 of *EuropeActive's Foundations for Exercise Professionals* (Moody and Stevens 2015) for a summary of the 1RM testing protocol.

An alternative to directly testing a client's 1RM is to estimate it using a prediction equation. In addition to the formula found in Lombardi (1989), chapter 15 explains how to use Brzycki's formula (1998) to calculate a client's 1RM from a testing protocol involving lighter loads and more repetitions than a 1RM.

See table 11.9 for more details about how to apply the health-related fitness component assessment model described in table 11.1 to muscular strength testing.

Table 11.9 Three Levels of Assessment for Muscular Strength

Levels of assessment	Target client	Assessment procedures
Level 1	Clients concerned only with overall well-being and not concerned at all with performance	No assessment needed (but that does not mean that assessment is inappropriate)
Level 2	Clients somewhat concerned with gaining muscle mass or performing strength-related exercises or tasks	1RM prediction equations applied to all exercises
Level 3	Clients highly focused on gaining muscle mass or on strength-related exercises or tasks; high-performance athletes	Directly measured 1RM on all appropriate exercises

Flexibility

Like many health-related components of fitness, a client's ability to move their body through a certain range of motion is specific to the joint or joints and the muscle–tendon complex being assessed (Mac-Dougall et al. 1991). Personal trainers can use a variety of techniques and tools to test a client's flexibility, such as visual observations, a sit-and-reach box, handheld goniometer, a smartphone app and measuring sticks of varying lengths.

The sit-and-reach test shown in chapter 19 of *EuropeActive's Foundations for Exercise Professionals* (Moody and Stevens 2015) assesses the flexibility of a client's lower back and posterior muscles of the lower body. To test a client's upper body flexibility, a personal trainer can choose the back scratch test (Heyward 2010).

Back Scratch Test

Protocol

- Allow the client to warm up.
- Have the client raise their right arm and position it next to the right side of the head with the elbow flexed and the palm of the right hand on the upper back behind the head. Simultaneously have the client reach up behind their back with the left hand and place the back of the left hand against their back.
- Direct the client to try to overlap the fingers of both hands as far as possible (figure 11.4a). For some clients, the fingers may not touch, leaving a gap between them.
- Measure the length of the overlap of the fingers (or the space between the hands) to the nearest centimetre (about .5 in.; figure 11.4b).
- If the client's fingers overlap, record the distance as a positive number; if there is a gap, record the distance as a negative number. A zero score is given when the fingertips touch.

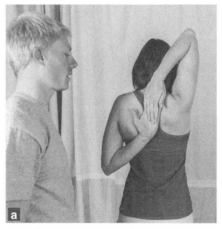

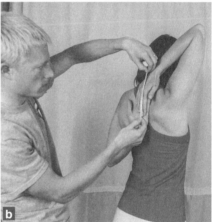

Figure 11.4 Back scratch test.

- Perform the test two more times and calculate the average distance.
- Switch the arm positions and repeat the test with the client's left arm next to the left side of the head and the right arm behind the back.

Advantages

- Easy to set up and administer
- Minimal equipment needed
- Can be conducted in nearly any location

Disadvantages

- Requires an administrator to properly perform the measurement
- Movements take place at several joints, so it is difficult to pinpoint one joint's range of motion.

Conclusion

The health and fitness assessment is one of the greatest tools a personal trainer can use to help a client reach high standards of success. The process promotes three vital goals: It helps assure clients' safety by assessing individual exercise-related risk and readiness, it provides data that can be used for building a comprehensive and highly individualised exercise programme and it allows personal trainers to monitor progression of all assessed health and fitness variables to objectively determine and report the success of the exercise programme. When a health and fitness assessment is consistently and effectively implemented, it can be a rewarding experience for both the client and the personal trainer.

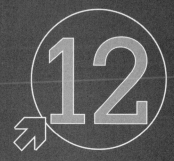

Psychological Aspects of Personal Training

Chris Beedie

The key mechanism of success in this field is the degree to which a personal trainer is conversant in and skilled with the principles of behaviour modification. That is, over and above being an expert in their specific scientific or professional discipline, personal trainers should also know how to use that knowledge to change their clients' lives. In short they can not only say *what* a client should do, but also identify *how* that client should do it. The aim of this chapter is to introduce the principles of behaviour modification as they apply to personal training and to present three simple tools that personal trainers can use to bring about desired outcomes reliably and predictably. The chapter should be read in conjunction with chapter 18 of *EuropeActive's Foundations for Exercise Professionals*.

Role of Psychology in Personal Training

Essentially this chapter is about psychology. At one level psychology is the science of mind and behaviour. Researchers in psychology seek to observe and explain links between mind and behaviour, as well as connections among these variables and diverse phenomena such as health, criminality, skill acquisition and educational achievement. At another level applied psychology uses the findings of research and of various psychological theories and models with the intention of bringing about changes in the mind and behaviour of the patient or client. In one form or another applied psychology is a feature of many domains of professional practice, from medicine, health and education to law enforcement, military service and sport performance.

The core role of personal trainers is to bring about meaningful change in the health, wellness and fitness status of their clients. This nearly always entails changes in both the client's mind (e.g., knowledge, beliefs, expectations and perceptions) and behaviour (e.g., improved movement frequency and quality, modified nutritional intake). A cursory glance at the role of the personal trainer demonstrates that most of the desired outcomes of training programmes depend on such modifications to the client's mind and behaviour. To be a good personal trainer, it is necessary to be a good psychologist.

However much confusion exists in media and society as to what 'doing psychology' actually means. The domain of applied psychology in fact spans everything from a mother using encouraging words to guide her child through their first attempt at crawling to the clinical psychologist helping a client through a serious mental condition such as depression or post-traumatic stress. It might be argued that mothers use common sense with no formal training, whilst clinical psychologists rely on several years of education and supervised clinical experience to guide their thinking and decisions.

In relation to the previous paragraph note that the level of applied psychology required in most personal training situations has far more in common with the former example (the mother) than the latter (the clinical psychologist). Although applied psychology for personal training requires a considered approach, a high degree of care and a genuine desire to help the client, it does not require either formal academic training or clinical experience in psychology. However all personal trainers must recognise that many of the conditions clients present with might require professional psychological or medical intervention (e.g., eating disorders, body image disorders, mood disorders). Personal trainers should always either refer or seek a professional opinion in any case in which they believe that the client may be experiencing a mental health problem (this is beyond the scope of this chapter; see, for example, Comer 2012 for details of conditions that fall into this category and their associated symptomology).

This chapter focuses on three key psychological processes in the context of personal training: goals and goal setting, beliefs and expectations, and emotions, stress and coping. Although other psychological variables might affect the processes and outcomes of fitness instruction, some knowledge of and skill with the management of these three factors is invaluable to most personal trainers.

Goals and Goal Setting

Goals motivate behaviour. The anticipation of an outcome motivates people to behave in a manner that will allow them to achieve this outcome. Personal trainers who can set appropriate goals will therefore likely have well-motivated clients, and a well-motivated client is more likely to succeed than a poorly motivated client. However the opposite is also true; poorly set goals are a significant factor in demotivation. Although a goal that is tangible, realistic and meaningful will likely positively affect behaviour, a goal that is intangible, unrealistic and not meaningful will not. A major reason that people come to personal trainers for help is that they have failed one or more times to succeed in fitness in the past, and a key reason for this failure is that they have often set poor goals that were intangible (e.g., 'I want to get a bit fitter.'), unrealistic (e.g., 'I want to run a marathon in 6 months time.') or not meaningful (e.g., 'I want to lose more weight than anyone else in the weight loss group.') (Siegert and Taylor 2004). The failure to achieve such goals leads to demotivation and often to relapse to previous behaviours. In such a very common scenario, the biggest effect a personal trainer can make is to help the client set appropriate goals and to subsequently monitor the client's process of achieving them. Table 12.1 uses the acronym SMART to guide trainers in crafting goals that are specific (S), measureable (M), achievable (A), regularly (R) reviewed and timed (T). This information is, to all intents, common sense. That is nothing in the content of this table should come as any surprise to anyone who has ever worked with clients in a fitness context.

The key component of the preceding table that clients tend to get wrong when left to their own devices is the balance between an achievable goal and a challenging one, a combination that describes the degree to which the goal is realistic. Many people either set goals that are too hard and unrealistic (e.g., 'I will lose 1 kilogram [2 pounds] per week for 4 months.') or make plans that are insufficient for achieving the desired outcome (e.g., 'I want to lose 13 kg [28 pounds] and will aim to exercise once a week.'). The task of a personal trainer is to negotiate a reasonable balance of what is possible and what is likely. For most people losing 1 kilogram of fat per week, although possible, is unlikely; that is, the client will need an energy deficit of 7,000 calories per week or 1,000 calories per day. This is perhaps possible if the person in question substantially both overeats and is overfat. However for most people a deficit of 1,000 calories per day would require a substantial change to both exercise and diet behaviour that they are unlikely to either practise or sustain.

Table 12.1 Goal Setting Using the SMART System

	Description	Bad example	Good example	Why is this a good example?
Specific	The goal must be a specific state that both the personal trainer and client understand.	'I want to be a fitter runner.'	'I want to be able to run without having to stop and walk every 5 minutes.'	The goal specifies what being a fitter runner means to the client. It is therefore specific and meaningful.
Measureable	The goal must have a specific quantity.	'I want to run farther than I can now.'	'I want to be able to run 5 km non-stop.'	It provides both the personal trainer and the client with a defined quantity of the goal to work towards. The client will also know when they have achieved it.
Achievable yet challenging	The goal must be sufficiently challenging to motivate the client but not so challenging as to demotivate them.	'I want to lose 10 kg (22 lbs) in 2 months.'	'I would also like to lose 1 kg (2 lbs) per month.'	Although the goal in the good example is certainly challenging, and if maintained over a year would lead to almost 13 kg of weight loss, it is still achievable in a well-designed exercise and diet programme *assuming that the client has that much fat to lose in the first place* (see table 12.2).
Regularly reviewed	The personal trainer must regularly check the client's progress towards the goal. If the client is moving too slowly or too fast, the personal trainer must modify the goal.	'We'll see how things go....'	'We will check your body weight and body mass every 4 weeks. We will also aim for you to be able to run 1 kilometre farther without stopping each month.'	Regular review periods allow the personal trainer to intervene and reset goals if progress is not as expected.
Timed	A timeline for goals allows the personal trainer to establish the process by which the client will achieve them.	'I'm going to just keep getting fitter.'	'I want to be able to run 5 km by June 30th.'	

In this context therefore the personal trainer and the client must agree not only on a certain goal but also on how that goal is to be achieved. For example, it is not good enough to say 'Let's aim for half a kilogram (1 pound) of weight loss per week' without stating exactly how the client will achieve this. That is, where are those calories going to come from? Reduced intake (diet), increased output (exercise) or a combination of the two? Weight loss does not happen by magic when a client begins to work with a personal trainer; it is the result of a considered balance of many factors monitored by the personal trainer. If clients realise that a set goal is not practicable, they will tend to blame either themselves for not being sufficiently motivated or the personal trainer for setting them up to fail. Either way, clients become demotivated, and their personal trainers have to work hard to get them back on track.

A goal plan that is well thought through and presented is a powerful tool in terms of both motivation and marketing. It provides a clear process for the personal trainer and the client to work from and shows the prospective client the likely scope of the process they are considering undertaking. The client shares what they want to achieve, and the personal trainer maps it out for them there and then. In most cases both enter into a negotiation that balances what the personal trainer believes the client will need to do and what the client says they are prepared to do. The outcome goal (i.e., the final level of weight loss, improved performance) is then renegotiated (table 12.2).

Perhaps the only component missing from the SMART model is process goals, that is, the goals that lead to the desired outcomes. For example, if the desired outcome is half a kilogram (1 pound) of fat loss per week, the process will require 500 kilocalories per day deficit, which would perhaps equate to one short exercise session per day with general food intake moderately reduced, or perhaps three longer sessions per week with slightly greater overall food reduction.

Beliefs and Expectations

A large database of research findings in medicine and the social sciences attests to what are termed *belief effects*. A belief effect is an outcome driven purely by the belief that a treatment has been received (Beedie et al. 2012). Belief effects have been reported in domains such as health, educational achievement and human performance and have been variously labelled the placebo effect, the Hawthorne effect and the Pygmalion effect (McCarney et al. 2007). In most cases these effects are explained by simple changes in behaviour brought about by the intervention; for example patients might take better care of themselves when they are being treated, athletes might try

Table 12.2 Sample Goal-Setting Process

	Goal	Specific and measureable	Achievable yet challenging	Process goals	Timed	Reviewed
	Fat loss	Client is currently 11 kg (25 lbs) overweight. A weight loss of 9 kg (20 lbs) is therefore reasonable and likely achievable.	3,500 calories deficit per week/500 calories per day	Increase physical activity (250kcals/day) Decrease intake of high energy foods (250kcals/day)	Goal achieved in approximately 6 months	Monthly review of body mass and body composition (to ensure that weight lost is mostly fat)
Notes		The goal must be both physiologically possible and safe. A 63.5 kg (140 lb) client with 15% body fat who wants to lose 4.5 kg (10 lbs) will either finish the process with extremely low fat mass or having lost lean body tissue, or will not finish the process at all. None of these outcomes is desirable for most clients; exceptions may include weight category athletes and other special populations.		Process goals are more controllable than outcome goals. However process goals must also be SMART.	Some flexibility around this time period will allow for unanticipated problems, such as illness or injury, and provide spare time if progress towards the goal is slower than expected. In relation to time frames, it is best to under-promise and overdeliver.	If the review shows either insufficient positive changes or any undesirable changes, the personal trainer must reset the process goals.

harder when they believe they have greater levels of physical capacity than is the case and students might work harder when they believe that they are more gifted than other students. Whatever the specific mechanisms, beliefs are powerful.

Most people who enter into an exercise programme do so with a set of beliefs about the likely results of that programme. A person new to exercise or diet might expect an almost magical transformation as the result of relatively little effort, whilst someone who has tried to exercise to lose weight several times might expect very little change despite a lot of hard work and personal investment. It is likely that both expectations are false. The former may be the result of a naive view of the rate of exercise-induced adaptation, and the latter possibly the result of previous failure that itself might have been the result of naive views of exercise. Either way beliefs, like goals, tend to affect motivation and therefore behaviour (Anshel 2014). Put simply if a client believes that exercising for 30 minutes a day and eating three fewer desserts per day will result in a predictable weight loss of around 230 to 450 grams (.5 to 1 pound) per week, they are more likely to engage positively with both processes than if they do not believe the process will be successful. As suggested previously some theories of the placebo effect suggest that what can appear to be a quite dramatic positive response to sham treatments (in medicine and beyond) simply results from the expectations of the person concerned, leading them to generally engage in more positive health behaviours.

A simple method that personal trainers can use to modify and reinforce beliefs includes the four sources of efficacy information (table 12.3). The confidence a person has in either a specific process or their ability to engage with that process has been labelled *self-efficacy* by psychologists. Self-efficacy is the degree of confidence a person has that they will achieve a specific goal (Weinberg and Gould 2011). Self-efficacy, like goal setting, is a relatively straightforward process, which personal trainers can implement easily, but which is often a very powerful motivational tool.

Research in psychology has suggested that people high in self-efficacy tend to set more challenging goals and to pursue those goals more vigorously than do people low in self-efficacy. On this basis, increasing clients' self-efficacy in relation to exercise, diet and lifestyle changes is likely to increase their motivation in all three. The preceding table shows the four main sources of efficacy information. The most powerful of these is personal experience, which makes intuitive sense given that we tend to base our expectations of the future on our experience of the past. However the majority of clients who arrive at the gym needing help will either lack personal

Table 12.3   Sources of Efficacy Information

Source of efficacy information	Description	Example	Strategies that can be used to implement the information
Previous performance	What the client has done previously	The client has successfully lost weight in the past (of course, if this is not the case, the personal trainer will need to either use one of the following strategies or help the client counter beliefs about previous experience).	Positive previous experience (positive self talk): 'I've done it before, I can do it again.' Negative previous experience (countering and positive self-talk): 'OK, it didn't work last time, but that doesn't mean it won't work this time.'
Vicarious experience	What someone similar to the client has done in the past	One of the personal trainer's previous clients of similar age and fitness successfully lost the required amount of weight in the past.	Countering or reframing: 'If people similar to me have done it, there's no reason why I shouldn't be able to.'
Verbal persuasion	The content of communication between the personal trainer and client	The personal trainer constantly reminds the client that they have the characteristics and opportunity to be successful.	Positive self-talk: 'My trainer believes I have the strength and commitment to do it, and she's an expert.'
Physiological and emotional arousal	The interpretation of the client's physiological and emotional symptoms	The personal trainer helps the client interpret pain as a sign that they are pushing their body beyond its current capacity, and therefore are likely to experience positive adaptation. Negative physiological symptoms are therefore reinterpreted as positive signs.	Reframing: 'Muscle soreness during exercise is a sign that I'm doing it right and that the muscles will adapt and get stronger.' Reframing: 'I get anxious at the thought of what I have to do, but that anxiety makes it even more rewarding when I've done it.'

experience of success in relation to exercise or dietary regulation or perhaps have negative experiences of these. Therefore many personal trainers spend a lot of time either *reframing* their client's experiences (essentially turning a negative experience into a potentially positive one), countering a client's faulty beliefs (e.g., challenging the basis for an attitude such as 'I'm just not cut out for exercise'), or using the *vicarious* experiences of others to instil a set of positive expectations. They might also employ verbal persuasion (e.g., the use of positive terminology and imagery when discussing ostensibly negative processes) and train the client to reinterpret their physiological or emotional signals in a more motivational manner (figure 12.1).

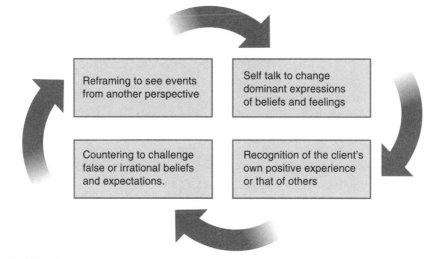

Figure 12.1 Process of modifying and reinforcing beliefs.

Emotions, Stress and Coping

Due to their proximity to clients, personal trainers must understand the relevance of emotions and stress and know how to cope with them during exercise sessions.

Emotion

Emotions play a big role in exercise. The emotions most commonly associated with exercise are generally positive, such as the endorphin high following a session or the euphoria and elation experienced at a personal best performance. However clients trying to adopt exercise habits often experience negative emotions such as anxiety, depression and guilt. Thus personal trainers must both understand how these emotions might influence their client's progress and know how to help the client cope when emotions take over.

Emotions, as their name suggests (e-*motion*), are psychological processes strongly associated with movement. Many researchers agree that emotions evolved to facilitate behaviour that helped us cope with stressors in an ever-changing and often dangerous world. An often-cited example of the relationship among emotion, stress and movement is the fight-or-flight response associated with the emotions of anger and fear, respectively. In both cases a perception and appraisal of some stressor in our environment stimulates a physiological and behavioural response that in anger tends to make us want to get closer to the cause and deal with it (fight), and which in fear tends to make us want to get as far away from the cause as possible (flight). Emotion tends to bias behaviour. However not all of these biases are obvious to either the personal trainer or the client. For example, whilst emotions such as excitement might be both motivational and easy to observe, other emotions might have more complex relationships with behaviour. For example, depression about life might generally lead to overeating, guilt about poor diet might lead to obsessive exercising and anger about work-related issues might lead to exercising at an inappropriate intensity. Each of these could be barriers to clients achieving their goals.

Although emotion is complex, some simple generalisations can be made about emotion in the exercise domain. First people tend to experience positive emotions such as happiness and contentment when they achieve a goal. Second people who experience positive emotions resulting from maintaining changes in exercise or diet are more likely to experience high self-efficacy and are therefore more likely to persist with these behaviours (and as long as they have new and challenging goals to pursue, this cycle will tend to keep people motivated and feeling good over many months and years). Of course the opposite is true: People who fail to achieve goals often experience low self-efficacy and, as a result, do not persist with behaviour change towards long-term goals. In such scenarios people often adopt behaviours to help themselves feel better in the short term, for example, use of alcohol, nicotine and other substances, poor dietary choices such as high-sugar or high-fat foods and inappropriate modes or intensities of exercise. Although there is nothing wrong with such behaviours in themselves, for many people it is their previous reliance on such behaviours that contributed to their failure to achieve goals and caused them to seek a personal trainer in the first place. Mechanisms to deal with emotions are addressed in the following section Coping With Stress and Negative Emotions.

Coping With Stress and Negative Emotions

Stress is a word that is often used in the exercise and health context. It is fair to say that there is a popular misconception that exercise and other health-related strategies will automatically reduce stress. However stress is a difficult idea to quantify because what one person finds stressful another person does not. Furthermore, in physiological terms, exercise is a source of stress. In this context it is important to consider that no matter how beneficial they may be, exercise, nutritional restriction and meaningful lifestyle modification are often perceived as sources of stress by the client, even if they are normal behaviour to the personal trainer. If this stress is perceived by the client to be at too high a level, either in itself (which is rare unless we are talking about elite athletes) or in combination with other stressors such as those related to work, family and finance, it is easy for a potentially positive process to become a negative one. Not only does this stress add to those stressors already being experienced, but the effect of the physiological symptoms of stress on endocrine and immune function often lead to poor adaptation to exercise and even regression (i.e., the client becomes less fit), to reduced resistance to infection and to ongoing negative emotional states such as low-level depression or free-floating anxiety (this collection of symptoms is often termed *overtraining syndrome* when experienced by elite athletes). Thus if even positive factors can be construed as stressful, it is important that the client has some mechanisms for coping with them.

The personal trainer works with the client for no more than a few hours per week. During that time the potential effects of stress and negative emotions are controlled by the personal trainer. However there are a considerably greater number of hours per week that clients will have to cope for themselves. Therefore personal trainers need three things: first a repertoire of coping strategies for a range of scenarios, second the ability to recognise which of these will work for a specific client in a specific context, and third the ability to train clients to use the coping strategies.

Although many models of coping have been proposed, it is fair to split coping strategies into two broad categories, *problem focused* and *emotion focused.* Problem-focused strategies are adopted in situations in which the problem can be dealt with. Emotion-focused strategies are employed once the problem has occurred and in situations where the potential for a negative emotional response and associated behavioural relapse is present. For example a client who is trying to reduce alcohol intake (and let's not forget that for many weight-loss clients, alcohol constitutes not only a distraction from more positive behaviours but also a substantial component of their daily energy surplus), a problem-focused coping strategy might be to drink a spritzer (50 percent wine, 50 percent soda water) at a dinner instead of wine alone. Alternatively clients could order a glass of water with every glass of wine. Both strategies tend to reduce the overall level of wine drunk at dinner, the total calories that day and perhaps the potential negative aspects of alcohol intake the following day (especially if a high level of alcohol is likely to have a negative effect on a scheduled exercise session in the morning).

However if the client goes to a dinner and fails to stick to their planned level of wine intake, they may wake the next morning experiencing any of a number of negative emotions, for example, guilt, shame, anxiety and anger. Although anger might promote a hard training session (that might not be the best idea with a hangover), none of these emotions is likely to make the client feel good about themselves, and several might predict reduced self-efficacy (e.g., 'I thought I could do this but I can't.' or 'I'm never going to lose this weight.'), which itself might predict poor adherence to exercise and to other behaviours aimed at the client achieving their goals. So the clients need strategies not only for preventing the problem occurring, but also for limiting the negative effect of negative emotions, that is, emotion-focused coping strategies (table 12.4).

Conclusion

This chapter provides a basic introduction to the role of psychology in fitness personal training. It is based on three specific areas: setting goals, modifying and reinforcing beliefs and coping with stress and negative emotions. These three aspects of psychology represent only a tiny percentage of the total number of psychological factors that might affect a person during their journey from novice client to self-coaching and self-monitoring regular exerciser. They do however provide three very simple and relatively powerful techniques by which the personal trainer might make the process shorter, more predictable and less stressful for the client. In fact they can be summarised in just a few short sentences:

1. Ensure that all the goals set by the client conform to the SMART model. That is, goals should be specific, measureable, achievable yet challenging (i.e., realistic), regularly reviewed and timed.

2. Ensure that the client holds positive beliefs about the likely outcomes of the exercise process. If they do, use efficacy information to reinforce these positive beliefs and expectations. If they do not, use efficacy information to modify these beliefs.

3. Ensure that the client is able to cope with the stress and negative emotional responses that might be part and parcel of an exercise programme and that are certainly part and parcel of everyday life for most people.

Table 12.4 Problem- and Emotion-Focused Coping Strategies

	Problem-focused strategy (used to reduce the likelihood of a potential problem)	Emotion-focused strategy (used to stop catastrophic thinking resulting from a setback such as 'I'm just not cut out for exercise.')
Smoking	'I won't socialise with people who smoke when I'm also having an alcoholic drink and might be more tempted than usual.'	'Having smoked a cigarette doesn't make me a smoker, just someone who had a cigarette.'
Sugary snacks	'I will not keep my problem foods in the house.' 'I will buy only what is on my shopping list (and I will not put doughnuts on my shopping list).' 'I won't go to the supermarket hungry.' 'I will have standby healthy snack foods in the house or at work to prevent me succumbing to chocolate.'	'I will offset the extra energy by either doing one extra exercise session or by adding 10 minutes to the next three sessions.' 'The fact that I noticed I'd eaten the chocolate shows how much I've improved, and that gives me confidence.'
Missed exercise session	'I will write every session in my diary so that I can't inadvertently book a conflicting appointment.'	'I will try to do the session at another time or will add a little extra time to each session next week to make up the session lost.'
Lack of motivation or tiredness	'If I don't feel up to going to the gym, I will still go for a walk just to keep the exercise habit going.' 'I will arrange to meet at least one of my friends at the class so that I feel I'm not just letting myself down if I don't go.'	'Missing a session or two isn't a problem in the big picture. However next time I miss a scheduled session I'll take a short walk just to keep the habit going, no matter how tired or unmotivated I feel.'
Injury	'If my shin splints flare up again I will use the bike or swim and will ask my trainer to write this into my programme.'	'I started the session, and it was too painful to continue. I will see a physiotherapist as soon as possible and find alternative exercises until the injury clears up.'
Illness	'If I start to feel slightly unwell I will stop training and help my body fight the infection. That way, I will lose the fewest possible days training.'	'I trained when I was feeling slightly ill and now it's got worse. I will simply have to accept that training is unlikely to be beneficial now and that I am more likely to recover quickly if I rest and take things easy.'

Note that the coping strategies are presented in the form of a positive self-talk statement made by the client, which is the way I have always preferred to train my clients to use both problem- and emotion-focused strategies. There are, of course, a number of different methods by which these can be deployed.

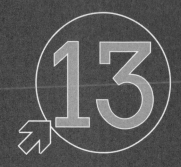

Nutrition

Fernando Naclerio

Robert Cooper

Proper nutrition is an important consideration for optimising health and quality of life. According to the National Centre for Health statistics, of the 10 leading causes of death, 5 of these (coronary heart disease and generalised arthrosclerosis, cancer, stroke, diabetes and kidney disorders) have been associated with dietary excess or imbalance. By following good nutritional practice people can maintain their health and enjoy an active lifestyle. Personal trainers are responsible for helping clients learn appropriate nutrition behaviours. This chapter describes the basic guidelines for nutrition, caloric intake, dietary habits, eating patterns and gaining or losing weight.

Energy Requirement

Adequate dietary guidelines should be based on the energy balance determined from the caloric expenditure and intake from the food (Manore and Thompson 2000). The energy requirement is determined by resting metabolic rate (RMR), the thermic effect of food and physical activity. Each of these factors can be affected directly or indirectly by age, genetics, body size, body composition, environmental temperature, physical activity demand (sedentary, active or athlete) and caloric intake.

Resting metabolic rate, a measure of the calories required for maintaining normal body functions such as respiration, cardiac function and thermoregulation, accounts for 65 to 75 percent of total daily energy expenditure. For children and adolescents growth also results in increased energy needs. Other factors that can raise RMR are an increase in lean body tissue, abnormal body temperature, menstrual cycle and hyperthyroidism. Factors that decrease RMR are low caloric intake, loss of lean tissue and hypothyroidism. Additionally normal genetic differences in metabolism can account for variations of 10 to 20 percent (Reimers 2008).

The thermic effect of food observed after eating is the increase in energy expenditure above the RMR due to digestion, absorption, metabolism and storage of food in the body. This effect can represent around 7 to 10 percent of the total energy requirement (Reimers 2008).

Physical activity is quite variable among different people. The number of calories expended through physical activity change depending on several factors, such as intensity, volume, duration or frequency and type of activities.

Estimating Energy Expenditure

The methods of measuring or estimating energy expenditure range from direct but complex measurements of heat production (direct calorimetry) to relatively simple indirect metabolic measurements (indirect calorimetry), and from expensive stable isotope tracer methods (doubly labelled water) to relatively cheap and convenient rough estimates (heart rate monitoring and accelerometry). However, due to individual differences, it becomes very difficult to accurately estimate energy expenditure, especially in sedentary older adults whose RMR tends to decrease approximately 2 to 3 percent every 10 years after 30 years old (Poehlman and Melby 1998).

Calculating Energy Needs

From a practical point of view, although not very accurate, it can be possible to estimate daily caloric (energy) needs using specific formulas (Kleiner 2008). The two prediction equations considered to most closely estimate energy expenditure are the *Cunningham equation* (Cunningham 1980) and the *Harris–Benedict equation* (Harris and Benedict 1918). Because the Cunningham equation requires that lean body mass be known, sport dieticians typically use the Harris–Benedict equation, which uses age (years), body mass (kg) and height (cm) to predict RMR:

Women: 655.1 + (9.56 × mass) + (1.85 × height) – (4.68 × age)

Men: 66.47 + (13.75 × mass) + (5.0 × height) – (6.76 × age)

Once RMR has been calculated, it is multiplied by the corresponding physical activity (PA) factor to estimate total energy expenditure. To get a relatively accurate estimate, personal trainers should interview clients about their daily activities (e.g., eating, sleeping, shopping, reading, walking, stair climbing) as well as their sport or specific exercise activities over a time period of a week (table 13.1; Kleiner 2008). Because Harris–Benedict equations published in 1918 were based on a population of 136 men (27 ± 9 years and 64 ± 10 kg) and 103 women (33.1 ± 14 years and 56.5 ± 11.5 kg), in order to reduce inaccurate estimates of RMR, further predictive equations based on the doubly labelled water technique have been developed:

Women: RMR = 354-6.91 × age (in years)
+ [PA × 9.36 × mass (in kg) + 726 × height (in meters)]

Men: RMR = 662-9.53 × age (years)
+ [PA × 15.91 × mass (in kg) + 539.6 × height (in meters)]

Table 13.1 Physical Activity (PA) Factors for Adults (>19 Years Old)

Activity level	Activity description	Total energy expenditure
Sedentary	Sitting and standing; no vigorous activities (mainly office work, driving, cooking)	1.0–1.39
Low activities	In addition to the activities of sedentary lifestyles, 30 minutes of daily moderately intensive activities equivalent to walking 3.2 km (2 miles) in 30 minutes. This category includes most office workers who exercise outside of work.	1.4–1.59
Active	In addition to the activities of the low-activity lifestyle, an additional 3 hours per day of activities such as cycling 16–19.2 km/hour (10–12 mph), stair climbing, walking 6.4 km/hour (4 mph), running 9.6 km/hour (6 mph). This category includes people with active jobs or clients who do 3 hours of planned vigorous exercise each day.	1.6–1.89
Very active	This category includes full-time athletes, unskilled labourers, members of the military and those on active duty, steel workers.	1.9–2.5

Recommended Dietary Intakes

The primary goal of the first recommended dietary allowance (RDA) in 1941 was to prevent diseases caused by nutrient deficiencies in populations such as children or members of the military, rather than to determine nutrient needs for individuals. Statistically speaking RDAs would prevent deficiency diseases in 97 percent of a population, but there was no scientific basis that RDAs would meet the needs of a single person (Jeukendrup and Gleeson 2010). Nowadays RDA guidelines focus on preventing the incidence of diet-related chronic disorders such as heart disease, diabetes, hypertension and osteoporosis, and they have been adapted to specific needs according to sex, age and special situations such as pregnant and lactating women. The dietary reference intake (DRI) is the new standard for nutrient recommendations that can be used to plan and assess diets for healthy people.

The DRI is a new concept that considers the following references or standard values:

- *Estimated average requirement (EAR):* This is the nutrient intake value that is estimated to meet the requirement for half of the healthy people in a group.

- *Recommended dietary allowance (RDA):* This value is based on the EAR. It is the daily dietary intake level that is sufficient to meet the nutrient requirement of 97 to 98 percent of all healthy people in a specific group.

- *Adequate intake (AI):* This value is used when an RDA cannot be determined. It is a recommended daily intake level based on an observed or experimentally determined approximation of nutrient intake for a group (or groups) of healthy people.

- *Tolerable upper intake level (UL):* This is the highest level of daily nutrient intake that is likely to pose no risks of adverse health effects to almost all people in the general population. As intake increases above the UL, the risk of adverse effects also increases.

Healthy Eating Patterns

A balanced diet is appropriate for athletes as well as for those in the general population (Brooks et al. 2004). The physiological needs of athletes and active people often require diets that are quite different from that of a sedentary person (Reimers 2008). The optimal diet for a client depends on many intrinsic factors, such as age, body size, sex and genetics as well as other external variables such as their type and level of physical activity and performance. When working with athletes personal trainers should change diet strategy depending on the client's specific goals for each training period or the competition demands associated with each specific sport, with the best diet being one that is individualised (Naclerio and Figueroa Alchapar 2011).

How Dietary Intake Influences Health

For optimising body composition, the most important diet variables to control are energy intake and energy expenditure (Rodriguez et al. 2009). People need to consume amounts of nutrients that will provide enough energy for health and help them maintain an adequate range of body weight and body composition. Dietary factors related to over- or undereating, particularly at different life stages, are poorly understood (La Bounty et al. 2011). Dietary fat has long been presumed to be a leading cause of weight gain. However other dietary composition factors, such as fibre, energy density, or glycemic index and load (Naclerio and Figueroa Alchapar 2011) as well as eating frequency, snacking and skipping meals, have been suggested to significantly influence energy regulation, body weight and body composition (La Bounty et al. 2011).

Overeating

Reduced total caloric intake has been shown to promote health benefits in overweight and normal-weight adults. Some of these benefits are reduced blood pressure, C-reactive protein (CRP), fasting plasma glucose and insulin, total and LDL cholesterol and atherosclerotic plasma formation (Manore and Thompson 2000).

The quantity, volume and macronutrient composition of the meals can affect hunger and the feeling of satiety. Hunger has been recognised as a negative feeling that needs to be avoided in order to control appetite and anxiety (Naclerio and Figueroa Alchapar 2011). Eating large amounts of food that contain high-density carbohydrate, such as sugar, candy, baked goods or even pasta and rice have been shown to negatively affect metabolic control and to stimulate the feeling of hunger. Research has suggested that eating small meals frequently throughout the day may not only positively affect metabolic control and glucose and insulin levels, but may also affect gastric stretching and gastric hormones that control satiety (La Bounty et al. 2011). Eating more frequently has been shown to be a better approach for reducing glucose and insulin response at subsequent meals. Consuming 4 to 6 or even up to 10 (in athletes) moderate to small meals per day has shown to be a good eating pattern for controlling hunger and the amount of daily food intake (La Bounty et al. 2011). The best time to eat is before hunger pangs strike (Roberts 2000).

When total energy intake is maintained, frequently consuming small meals seems to improve lipid profile and decrease blood pressure, glucose kinetics and insulin responses (La Bounty et al. 2011). Conversely, although data are very limited about the effect of meal frequency on health and body composition, sedentary people who skip meals with the aim of decreasing caloric intake actually gain weight (Bellisle et al. 1997). A negative correlation between meal frequency and both BMI and waist-to-hip ratio has been seen, even after adjusting for under-reporters and dieters (Ruidavets et al. 2002).

Undereating

The newer concept of energy availability, defined as dietary intake minus exercise energy expenditure normalised to fat-free mass, is the amount of energy available to the body to perform all other functions after exercise training expenditure is subtracted (Rodriguez et al. 2009). Among active or athletic populations, some female athletes may consume less energy than they expend (Rodriguez et al. 2009). Low energy intake (e.g., 1,800 to 2,000 kilocalories per day or less) for female athletes is a major nutritional concern because a persistent state of negative energy balance can lead to weight loss, hinder endocrine function, compromise performance and negate the benefits of exercise or training (Rodriguez et al. 2009). With limited energy intake the body uses fat and lean tissue for fuel. Loss of lean tissue mass impairs power, strength and muscular endurance.

A considerable body of evidence suggests that a low availability of energy has serious consequences on a person's hormonal, immunological and health status. This is best demonstrated in the female athlete triad, where low energy availability, impaired menstrual status and poor bone health are inter-related (Burke et al. 2006). Many female athletes develop metabolic, reproductive and bone disruptions because they over-restrict their energy intake to lose body fat. Incremental changes in energy availability lead to a dose-dependent relationship between energy restrictions and metabolic and hormonal function; the threshold for maintenance of normal menstrual function in women is an energy availability of more than 30 kilocalories (125 kJ) per kilogram of fat-free mass. Male athletes who expose themselves to periods of low energy availability will likely also suffer from metabolic and reproductive disturbances. Long-term low-energy intake results in poor nutrient consumption; in particular low levels of micronutrients may result in metabolic dysfunctions associated with nutrient deficiencies as well as in lowered RMR (Rodriguez et al. 2009).

Clients must not follow overly restricted diets in order to achieve their desired body composition (La Bounty et al. 2011). Increasing meal frequency under hypocaloric conditions may have anticatabolic effects (protection of muscle mass) even if the weight loss could be the same compared to that achieved on a low-frequency meal plan (Iwao et al. 1996).

In restricted caloric diets the protein content of total caloric intake seems to be a very important factor in terms of preserving lean tissue. Frequent feedings with higher protein content (15% vs. 10%) may reduce nitrogen losses during periods of hypocaloric intake (La Bounty et al. 2011). In order to protect skeletal muscle and optimise muscle protein balance, clients will likely need to adjust protein intake on a per meal basis (Børsheim et al. 2002). Protein synthesis in skeletal muscle may be optimal when clients consume approximately 20 to 30 grams of high-quality protein or 10 to 15 grams of essential amino acids per meal (Dangin et al. 2003; Bohé et al. 2003). Equal distribution of protein over all of the meals in a day seems to result in greater protein synthesis and muscle mass when compared to an unequal distribution of protein with lower amounts consumed at breakfast and lunch and higher amounts at dinner. However if the quantity of protein provided in each meal increases to an optimal amount (15 grams per meal), along with increasing the meal frequency from 3 meals a day to 5 or 6, it will be possible to establish a positive influence between meal frequency and protein status. Therefore when the amount of protein ingestion is enough to optimise protein synthesis, increased meal frequency may positively affect protein status.

Micronutrient Deficiency and Health

To minimise risk of micronutrient deficiencies all clients, including athletes, should consume diets that provide at least the RDA for all micronutrients (Rodriguez et al. 2009).

Vitamins

Vitamins are organic compounds that cannot be synthesised by the body and therefore must be obtained through the diet. Vitamins are required in small amounts by the body for many essential physiological processes, such as energy production, antioxidant functions and muscle repair. Often considered accessory nutrients, vitamins do not supply energy. They serve as basic building units for other compounds and contribute substantially to the body's mass.

Thirteen different vitamins have been isolated, analysed, classified and synthesised. Recommended intake levels have been established for these vitamins. Vitamins are classified as either *fat soluble* (vitamins A, D, E and K) or *water soluble* (vitamin C and the B complex vitamins: vitamin B_6 [pyridoxine], vitamin B_1 [thiamine], vitamin B_2 [riboflavin], niacin [nicotinic acid], pantothenic acid, biotin, folic acid and vitamin B_{12} [cobalamin]).

Water-soluble vitamins disperse in the body's fluids without appreciable storage, with the excess voided in urine. If the diet regularly contains less than 50 percent of the recommended values for water-soluble vitamins, marginal deficiencies may develop within 4 weeks.

Fat-soluble vitamins are stored in the body's fatty tissues. They do not require daily intake. In fact symptoms of a fat-soluble vitamin insufficiency may not appear for years. However a prolonged inadequate intake of a particular vitamin can trigger symptoms of vitamin deficiency and lead to severe medical complications. For example symptoms of thiamine deficiency occur after only 2 weeks on a thiamine-free diet, and symptoms of vitamin C deficiency appear after 3 or 4 weeks. At the other extreme an overdose of the fat-soluble vitamins A, D, E and K (although very uncommon) can produce hair loss, irregularities in bone formation, foetal malformation, haemorrhage, bone fractures, abnormal liver function and ultimately death.

Minerals

Approximately 4 percent of the body's mass consists of 22 mostly metallic elements collectively called *minerals*. Minerals are inorganic elements that provide structure in forming bones and teeth. They help to maintain normal heart rhythm, muscle contractility, neural conductivity and acid–base balance, and help to regulate cellular metabolism by becoming part of enzymes, hormones that modulate cellular activity and vitamins. They combine with other chemicals (e.g., calcium phosphate in bone and iron in the *heme* of haemoglobin) or exist singularly (e.g., free calcium in body fluids). In the body *trace minerals* are those required in amounts of less than 100 milligrams a day, and *major minerals* are required in amounts 100 milligrams daily or more.

No difference exists between a vitamin or mineral obtained naturally from food and a vitamin produced synthetically. Manufacturers gain huge profits in advertising micronutrients as 'natural' or 'organically isolated', yet such vitamins or minerals are chemically identical to those synthesised in the laboratory.

Fads and Popular Diets

Fad diets are the kind of regimens where you eat a very restrictive diet or an unusual combination of foods for a short period of time in order to lose weight. In many cases it becomes very difficult to keep to the regimen. When people stop fad diets they usually regain the lost weight and even put on additional weight (Dansinger et al. 2005). Many different types of diet plans are appearing continuously on the market. The popular diets shown in figure 13.1 categorise the different strategies used based on nutritional emphasis (Naclerio and Figueroa Alchapar 2011).

No exact guidelines exist about the quantities of nutrients each type of diet must provide in order to be classified as a high- or low-fat (or high- or low-carbohydrate) programme. Moderate- or low-fat diets commonly provide no more than 30 percent of caloric energy from fat sources such as nuts, olives or fish oils. Extreme low-fat and high-carbohydrate diets include vegetarian diet, Pritikin diet (restricts fat consumption to 15 percent of total caloric intake) and Ornish diets (limits fat intake to 10 percent and emphasises the consumption of vegetables and fruits). These rich-carbohydrate diets are very restrictive in terms of fat, but they also provide a relatively low amount of protein that cannot be considered enough for more active people or athletic populations (Campbell et al. 2007; Ziegenfuss et al. 2010). Conversely low-carbohydrate diets such as Atkins, protein powder or Dukan diets are structured in stages. The carbohydrate

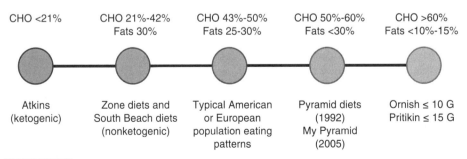

Figure 13.1 The continuum of popular diets ranging from low-carbohydrate to low-fat diets.

Reprinted from *Clinics in Sports Medicine,* Vol. 18(3). R.E. Riley, "Popular weight loss diets. Health and exercise implication," pgs. 691-701, copyright 1999, with permission from Elsevier.

intake is drastically reduced during the first phases (20 grams or even less per day) in order to stimulate rapid weight loss and control blood glucose and insulin concentrations. After the rapid weight loss phase, carbohydrate intake can further be increased to 90 grams per day (Atkins diet; Atkins 1998) or 1 gram of carbohydrate per gram of ingested protein for sedentary people or 1.3 grams for more active or athletic subjects (protein powder diet; Riley 1999).

Moderate-carbohydrate diets such as the Zone, Palaeolithic or South Beach diets recommend that around 40 percent of energy should come from carbohydrate sources, whilst the remaining 60 percent should be equally distributed between fat (30%) and protein (30%). The Zone diet is a low-calorie programme to help people lose weight based on the balance of carbohydrate, protein and fat consumed at every meal. This combination, together with the control of glycemic index and load of carbohydrate-rich food, allows for an optimal control of insulin–glucagon axis responses.

The *glycemic index* is how fast a defined amount (50 grams) of available carbohydrate enters the bloodstream as glucose (Wolever 2006). It is considered a qualitative indicator of carbohydrate's ability to increase blood glucose levels. However to understand how carbohydrate affects insulin responses, it is necessary to consider the *glycemic load*, which represents the amount of available carbohydrate per serving. It can be calculated by multiplying the amount of carbohydrate in a meal by the glycemic index value published in the international table of glycemic index (Foster-Powell et al. 2002; see also www.glycemicindex.com). A high glycemic load reflects a greater expected elevation in blood glucose and a greater insulin response (release) to that food. Consuming a diet with a high glycemic load on a regular basis has been associated with an increased risk for type 2 diabetes and coronary heart disease, whereas consuming a diet with a low glycemic index (focusing on food such as vegetables and some fruits) has been shown to improve metabolic profile, weight control and health (Wolever 2006).

According to supporters of the Zone diet the equilibrium between the insulin and glucagon significantly affects whether the essential fatty acid consumed in the diets is converted to good or bad eicosanoids (Sears and Lawren 1995). These substances are considered *master switchers* that control virtually all human body functions. Good eicosanoids are those related to vasodilatations and lipid mobilisation processes, whereas bad ones are more related to vasoconstriction and inflammation process. The Zone diet involves eating meals and snacks every 4 hours, with an energetic composition of 40:30:30 coming from carbohydrate, fat and protein, respectively.

Some authors have suggested that the Zone diet is relatively safe if the energy level is not restricted to less than 1,000 kilocalories per day (Riley 1999). However this strategy has not been well accepted for some athletes due to its relatively low level of carbohydrate compared to traditional recommendations, which are that carbohydrate should make up around 50 percent of the total caloric intake depending on the individual's athletic needs (Rodriguez et al. 2009).

Food Pyramid and MyPlate Dietary Plans

In April 2005 the U.S. government unveiled a new attempt to personalise the approach to help Americans choose a healthier lifestyle that balances nutrition and exercise. The colour-coded food pyramid, termed MyPyramid, combined with a complementary web site provided personalised guidelines for eating patterns. MyPyramid depicted a series of vertical colour bands of varying widths with the combined bands for fruits (red band) and vegetables (green band) occupying the greatest width, followed by grains (orange), with the narrowest bands occupied by fat, oils, meat and sugar. The MyPyramid guidelines advised consuming a varied but balanced diet rich in fruits and vegetables, cereals and whole grains, non-fat and low-fat dairy products, legumes, nuts, fish, poultry and lean meats. MyPyramid did not, however, emphasise fluid intake, nor did it give a clear recommendation about portion size or number for each group of food (Shugarman 2008). MyPyramid also did not consider the glycemic index and load of the carbohydrate-rich food, which is a more useful physiological approach than simply classifying a carbohydrate based on its chemical configuration (Naclerio and Figueroa Alchapar 2011). The protein groups involved both meats and beans; however beans are a source of carbohydrate that provides soluble and insoluble fibre rather than protein. With regard to fat, MyPyramid did not make any recommendations about essential Omega-3 fatty acids. The unsuccessful MyPyramid lead the U.S. government to develop a new strategy for promoting healthy eating patterns. The MyPlate icon (figure 13.2) emphasizes the fruits,

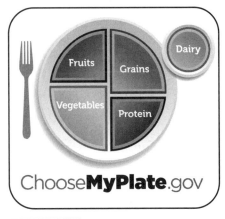

Figure 13.2   MyPlate.

USDA's Center for Nutrition Policy and Promotion.

vegetables, grains, protein foods and dairy groups. Although individuals can find very good advice and information by logging on to the website (www.choosemyplate.gov) MyPlate figures neglect the importance of fluids, which is perhaps the most important nutrient to consider, and oils. In general MyPlate provides practical information to individuals, health professionals, nutrition educators, and the food industry to help consumers build diets based on the prevalence of carbohydrates as the most important macronutrient.

Developing a Healthy, Balanced Way of Eating

No uniform criteria exist about the ideal macronutrient proportion for an optimal healthy diet programme. The positive outcomes achieved from low-carbohydrate or low-fat diets in terms of weight loss or control seem to be associated with a simultaneous physical activity programme rather than with the dieting strategy itself (Naclerio and Figueroa Alchapar 2011). Several studies have demonstrated that other than the total energetic caloric intake, the macronutrients in meals affect metabolic and hormonal responses after eating (Volek et al. 2005; Layman and Baum 2004; Layman et al. 2009). In fact moderate diets (40 percent carbohydrate) that maintain a protein–carbohydrate relationship of .6 to .75 have been shown to be more effective in controlling body weight and feeling of satiety in overweight and obese people than low-carbohydrate diets (Layman and Baum 2004; Layman et al. 2009; Layman et al. 2003). These effects have been associated with an increase of some appetite-inhibitory ketone bodies, reducing blood glucose and insulin levels (Volek et al. 2005; Fontani et al. 2005) and improving lipid profile (Layman et al. 2009).

When working with people from various backgrounds and cultures, it is important to remember that many different eating styles can equate to an adequate diet; there is no one right diet for all people. The guidelines of healthy diets should not include severe restrictive or deprivation measures, but rather educative programmes that lead participants into healthy eating behaviour and help them create good nutritional habits that they can maintain throughout their lives (Naclerio and Figueroa Alchapar 2011). The following recommendations can help both healthy active people and athletes accomplish adequate eating behaviours. These general recommendations can be adjusted by sport nutrition experts to accommodate the unique concerns of clients in terms of health, level of physical activity, sport, nutrient needs, food preferences and body weight and body composition goals.

1. Control the amount of food consumed at each meal, avoiding very large food intake before a long rest period (sleeping; Volpe 2006).

2. Minimise sugar intake. Sugar can be hidden in many food and drink products. Check the labels and choose lower-sugar alternatives. High sugar intake has been associated with increased blood triglyceride levels, which in turn are linked with insulin resistance. Sugar provides energy without providing any other worthy nutritional content.

3. More active people or athletes should consume a larger, hypercaloric meal with high-density carbohydrate (pasta, bread, rice or potatoes) within 4 hours after a training session, but not before sleeping (Ivy and Portman 2004). Carbohydrate recommendations for athletes range from 5 to 10 grams per kilogram of body weight for strength athletes or aerobic endurance athletes, respectively (Naclerio and Figueroa Alchapar 2011).

4. Protein requirements vary among people depending on activity levels. Sedentary people should aim to consume 1 gram of protein per kilogram of body weight, whilst athletes and more active people may find it beneficial to consume 1.2 to 1.7 grams of protein per kilogram of body weight for aerobic endurance athletes or 2 grams for strength athletes (Rodriguez et al. 2009; Campbell et al. 2007). Sources of protein include meat, poultry, fish and eggs. When selecting meat choose leaner cuts in order to limit intake of saturated fat (Naclerio and Figueroa Alchapar 2011).

5. Water is an essential nutrient. Fluid intake in less active or sedentary people should be around 30 millilitres per kilogram per day (2 to 3 L per day). After training athletes must drink 900 to 1,350 millilitres per kilogram of body weight lost (Rodriguez et al. 2009).

6. For athletes or regular exercise practitioners, postexercise dietary goals are to provide adequate fluids, electrolytes, energy and carbohydrate to replace muscle glycogen and ensure rapid recovery. Consuming approximately 1 to 1.5 grams of carbohydrate per kilogram of body weight during the first 30 minutes after a workout and again every 2 hours for 4 to 6 hours will be adequate to replace glycogen stores. Protein consumed after exercise provides amino acids for building and repairing muscle tissue (Rodriguez et al. 2009).

7. Total fat intake should match around 20 to 35 percent of total calories consumed (Rodriguez et al. 2009). This intake should be low in saturated fat with a balance of essential fatty acid from fish oils and monounsaturated sources (olive oils; Simopoulos 2002). Fat, which is a source of energy, fat-soluble vitamins and essential fatty acids, is important in an athlete's diet.

8. Consume milk and other dairy products in moderation to obtain the beneficial calcium but limit saturated fat (Williams 2005).

9. Moderate salt intake (do not exceed more than 6 grams per day; Williams 2005).

10. Ingest dietary supplements only if necessary to prevent deficiencies or match training requirements (Naclerio and Figueroa Alchapar 2011). In general no vitamin and mineral supplements are required if an athlete is consuming adequate energy from a variety of foods to maintain body weight. A multivitamin and mineral supplement may be appropriate when an athlete is dieting, habitually eliminating foods or food groups (as is generally observed in gymnastic or weight-class sports such as wrestling or boxing), is ill or recovering from injury, or if the athlete has a specific micronutrient deficiency. Single-nutrient supplements may be appropriate for a specific medical or nutritional reason (e.g., iron supplements to correct iron deficiency anaemia; Rodriguez et al. 2009).

11. Vegetarian athletes may be at risk for low intakes of energy, protein, fat and key micronutrients such as iron, calcium, vitamin D, riboflavin, zinc and vitamin B_{12} (Rodriguez et al. 2009). Consultation with a dietician is recommended in order to determine whether an athlete needs supplements to avoid these nutrition problems.

Tobacco, Alcohol and Caffeine

Avoiding bad habits such as smoking and excessive drinking contributes to a healthy lifestyle (Williams 2005). The American Surgeon General warns, 'There is no risk free level of exposure to tobacco smoke and no safe tobacco product (U.S. Department of Health and Human Services 2010). The World Health Organization estimates that the global yearly death toll as a result of tobacco use is currently 6 million (including exposure to second hand smoke) (Eriksen et al 2012). This is expected to rise to 7 million by 2020 and to more than 8 million a year by 2030 (U.S. Department of Health and Human Services, 2010). Additionally for every death caused by smoking, approximately 20 smokers are suffering from a smoking related disease For optimal health and exercise or sport performance the best solution is to not use tobacco products.

Moderate alcohol consumption is defined as an average daily consumption of one drink per day for women and up to two drinks per day for men. One drink is defined as 350 millilitres (~12 fluid oz.) of regular beer, 150 millilitres (5 fluid oz.) of wine or 45 millilitres (1.5 fluid oz.) of distilled spirits (DGAC 2010). This amount of alcohol has been shown to have a protective effect on coronary heart disease; however there are no guaranteed safe limits. Drinking too much can have many detrimental effects such as increased risk of cancer, liver disease, increased blood pressure and heart attack. In the UK it is recommended that men should not regularly drink more than four units of alcohol a day and women should not regularly drink more than three units of alcohol a day (DGAC 2010). Because most people do not drink every day, take this advice as a general average metric to be figured over the course of a week or month instead of an exact threshold of 'one drink per day for women or two drinks per day for men'. In addition strong evidence suggests that heavy consumption of four or more drinks a day for women and five or more drinks a day for men have harmful health effects. A number of situations and conditions call for the complete avoidance of alcoholic beverages (DGAC 2010).

Caffeine is found naturally in coffee beans, tea leaves, chocolate, cocoa beans and cola nuts, and it is added to carbonated beverages and non-prescription medicines. Depending on the preparation, 250 millilitres (1 cup) of brewed coffee contains between 60 and 150 milligrams of caffeine, instant coffee contains about 100 milligrams, brewed tea contains between 20 and 50 milligrams and caffeinated soft drinks contain about 50 milligrams (McArdle et al. 2011). Caffeine absorption by the small intestine occurs rapidly, reaching peak plasma concentrations between 30 and 120 minutes after ingestion. Caffeine exerts an influence on the nervous, cardiovascular and muscular systems. Its metabolic half-life ranges from 3 to 8 hours, which means that it clears from the body fairly rapidly, certainly after a night's sleep.

When consumed in low to moderate dosages (3 to 6 milligrams per kilogram of body weight, or around three cups of coffee), caffeine has been shown to be effective for enhancing sport performance in trained team sports and aerobic endurance and possibly in strength and power athletes. Higher dosage does not produce further enhancement. Its positive effects can also be extended to enhance vigilance during bouts of extended exhaustive exercise, as well as during periods of sustained sleep deprivation. Even if a high dosage of caffeine possibly stimulates diuresis at rest, the literature does not indicate any negative effect of caffeine on sweat loss and thus show a fluid balance during exercise that would adversely affect performance among athletes or exercising people (Goldstein et al. 2010). In general up to 200 milligrams of caffeine per day are considered fairly harmless, even if caffeine's effects and tolerances can vary among people (Williams 2005).

Fat and Lipoprotein

Dietary lipids serve as a carrier for the fat-soluble A, D, E and K vitamins. To meet recommended levels, 20 grams of dietary fat should be consumed daily. Thus voluntarily reducing lipid intake lowers the body's level of these vitamins, and may ultimately lead to vitamin deficiency. In addition dietary lipids delay the onset of hunger pangs and contribute to satiety after meals because the stomach takes about 3.5 hours to empty lipids into the digestive system. This explains why weight-loss diets that contain some lipids sometimes prove initially successful in blunting the urge to eat more than the extreme and heavily advertised fat-free diets. On the other hand excessive fat intake has been associated with glucose or lipid disorders and with increased risk of cardiovascular heart disease (McArdle et al. 2011). Although replacing saturated fat with carbohydrate has been a common public health recommendation, it is increasingly recognised that high carbohydrate intake can have the negative metabolic consequence of increasing triglycerides in sedentary or less active people (Reimers 2008).

Dietary Fat

The current recommendation to the general public is that fat should constitute 20 to 35 percent of total calories consumed (Reimers 2008). Less than 10 percent should come from saturated fat, 8 to 10 percent from monounsaturated fat and the other 8 to 10 percent from polyunsaturated fat. The latter should be ideally equally divided between Omega-3 and Omega-6 fatty acids (1:1 ratio; Simopoulos 2010). In order to increase the Omega-3 content of the diet, nutritionists should encourage that fat be consumed from natural sources, which include cold-water fatty fish (salmon, tuna or sardines) and oils such as canola, soybean, safflower, sunflower, sesame and flax.

Guidelines for dietary fat consumption for aerobic endurance athletes can be higher than those recommended for other populations. Research shows that during periods of heavy aerobic endurance training, in order to match the energetic demand of physical activity, increasing dietary fat from more than 30 percent to 40 or even 50 percent of calories does not negatively affect plasma lipids, and can positively influence performance (Leddy et al. 1997; Helge et al. 1998).

Cholesterol

Cholesterol can be manufactured from fat, carbohydrate or protein within the body; therefore there is little need to obtain dietary cholesterol, which is found only in animal products. When dietary cholesterol increases, endogenous production decreases and vice versa. The body needs cholesterol to produce steroid hormones, bile acids and vitamin D. Lipids are insoluble in water, and therefore are packaged up with protein to form a lipoprotein that enables transport in the blood stream.

The four types of lipoproteins are categorised according to their gravitational densities: chylomicrons, high density, low density and very low density. The liver and small intestine produce *high-density lipoprotein (HDL)*. Of the lipoproteins HDLs contain the greatest percentage of protein and the least total lipid and cholesterol, which helps them protect against heart disease. HDLs can be increased by exercise and weight loss. Degradation of a *very-low-density lipoprotein (VLDL)* produces a *low-density lipoprotein (LDL)*. The VLDL contains the greatest percentage of lipid. High levels of total cholesterol or unfavourable ratios of lipoproteins (HDL/LDL) are associated with increased risk of heart disease. Table 13.2 summarises the desired healthy blood lipid and lipoprotein levels.

Essential Fatty Acids (Omega-3 and Omega-6)

It is presently known that the essential fatty acids (FAs) of Omega-6 (especially linoleic acid and arachidonic acid [AA]) and Omega-3 (linolenic acid, eicosapentaenoic acid [EPA] and docosahexaenoic acid [DHA]) are essential for the formation of healthy cell membranes, proper development and growth, functioning of the brain and nervous system, as well as the production of hormones. Omega-3 has been shown to play a key role in the prevention and management of coronary disease, hypertension, diabetes, arthritis, cancer and other inflammatory and autoimmune conditions (Simopoulos 1991).

The modification of dietary patterns over the last 150 years has led to a change in FA consumption, with an increase in the consumption

Table 13.2 Lipid Blood Marker Recommendations

Blood marker	Desirable (mg/dl)	Limit (mg/dl)	High (mg/dl)
Total triglyceride	<150	200	>200
Total cholesterol	<200	240	>240
HDLs	40-50	<40 (low)	>60
LDLs	<100	160	>160
Ratio of total cholesterol to HDLs	3.6	4.5	>4.5
Ratio of LDLs to HDLs	2.5	3.5	>3.5
Ratio of total triglycerides to HDLs	2	4	>4

From Sears, B., & Lawren, B. 1995. *Enter the Zone.* New York: Regan Books; Naclerio, A.F. 2005. Nutrition and body weight control. In *Personal Training, Foundations and Applications,* edited by G.A. Jiménez. Barcelona: Inde (in Spanish).

of Omega-6 and a significant reduction in Omega-3 intake. This, in turn, has given rise to an imbalance in the ratio of Omega-6 to Omega-3, being now between 10 to 1 and 25 to 1, which is very different from the original 1:1 ratio of humans in the past (Simopoulos 2008; Simopoulos 2010). Omega-6 and Omega-3 FAs are not interchangeable in the human body. Studies with non-human primates and human newborns indicate that DHA and EPA are essential components for normal functional development of the brain and retina, particularly in premature infants.

The types of FAs available for cell membrane formation and synthesis depend on diet and endogenous metabolism of FAs. However the critical factor in the efficiency of fatty acids is not their absolute level, but rather the ratio between various groups of FAs. It is known that the relative amounts of Omega-6 and Omega-3 in the cell membrane are responsible for affecting cellular function because arachidonic acid (AA) competes directly with EPA for incorporation into cell membranes. A low ratio of AA to EPA has been proposed as an index of the beneficial effects of Omega-3s. Clinical studies indicate that cognitive performance improves with supplementation of Omega-3s along with a positive influence on mood and emotional state (Simopoulos 1991; Simopoulos 2010). These data suggest that the balance of Omega-6 and Omega-3 fatty acids is a very important factor to consider for homeostasis and normal development throughout the life cycle (Simopoulos 2008; Simopoulos 2010; Simopoulos 1991).

An approximate estimation of the consumption of Omega-3 FAs in Europe is .1 to .5 grams per day. This is higher than the estimated intake of DHA and EPA in the United States (.1–.2 grams/day), but low in comparison with the data corresponding to Japan (up to 2 grams/day), where fish is one of the most commonly consumed foods (Gómez Candela et al. 2011). Many countries have recommended daily EPA and DHA intake levels ranging from 500 milligrams per day in France to 1 to 2 grams per day in Norway. The World Health Organization recommends the consumption of between .3 and .5 grams per day, whilst the International Society for the Study of Fatty Acids and Lipids advocates 500 milligrams per day and the North Atlantic Treaty Organization recommends 800 milligrams per day. The European Food Safety Authority postulates that the amount of EPA and DHA required to lower triglyceride levels is 2 to 4 grams per day, and 3 grams per day to lower blood pressure (Gómez Candela et al. 2011). Taking all this into account, the recommended amounts and the ideal FA ratio must be adjusted according to the findings from additional research.

Safe and Effective Weight Loss and Gain

Optimising lean body mass and body fat requires manipulation of both daily exercise activities and dietary strategies. Only with this approach can clients reach a healthy body weight and composition.

Weight Loss Management

In order to help clients lose weight personal trainers should address caloric deficits through a combination of reducing nutritional intake and increasing energy expenditure through exercise. The estimated minimal level of body fat compatible with health is 5 percent for men and 12 percent for women; however optimal body fat percentages for an individual person may be much higher than these minimums, depending on their daily activity demands and goals (Rodriguez et al. 2009). In addition the ability to achieve and maintain minimal amount of body fat is largely genetic (Reimers 2008). During the first 4 to 12 weeks of a combined caloric restriction diet and exercise programme, novice or sedentary clients can both lose body fat and gain lean body mass; however it is unlikely that trained athletes who already possess a relatively low percentage of body fat can reduce overall body mass without losing some lean body mass. In general fit people find it very difficult to lose substantial amounts of body mass without losing lean tissue, particularly when following a caloric restriction diet (Reimers 2008).

If all of the expended kilocalories on the diet are applied to body fat loss, a deficit of 3,500 kilocalories will result in a fat loss of .45 kilograms (1 pound). The maximal recommended rate of fat loss per week is near 1 percent of body mass. This is an average of .5 to 1.0 kilograms (1.1 to 2.2 pounds) per week, and it represents a daily caloric deficit of approximately 500 to 1,000 kilocalories. Faster rates can lead to dehydration and loss of lean tissue, and may possibly negatively affect micronutrient status. In addition to the percentage of fat, the maximum weight loss rates (kg) will depend on the initial body weight. For example a 65-kilogram (143 pound) woman who needs to reduce her fat mass should not lose more than .65 kilograms (1.4 pounds) per week. Conversely a man who is 120 kilograms overweight can safely lose 1.2 kilograms (2.6 pounds), which represents 1 percent of his body weight. Gradual weight loss ensures that fat is predominantly lost and lean tissue preserved, whilst extremely rapid weight loss can result in lean tissue (muscle and water) being primarily lost rather than fat.

For sedentary people common guidelines for weight loss are to consume a total daily caloric intake of 1,000 to 1,200 kilocalories for women and 1,500 kilocalories for men. However for most active people and athletes, these levels are too low. Ideally, caloric intake should be individualised. From a practical point of view this is a very difficult task for the personal trainer. A good approach could be to periodically control the client's body composition, physical and cognitive performance, mood state and willingness to be active. These variables, together with the feelings of anxiety and depression, have been shown to be significantly sensitive, and to decrease as a consequence of severe dietary restrictions (Naclerio 2005).

Weight Gain Management

Conversely to gain weight, a well-designed combination of hyper-caloric diet and exercise programme is advisable (Rodriguez et al. 2009). Generally people attempt to gain weight for two basic reasons: to improve physical appearance or to enhance athletic performance. For weight gain in the form of muscle mass, a combination of diet and progressive resistance training is essential. However genetic predisposition, body type and compliance determine the athlete's progress. If all the extra calories consumed are used for muscle growth during resistance training, then about 2,500 extra kilocalories are required for each 0.5 kilogram (~1 pound) increase in lean tissue. Thus, 350 to 700 kilocalories above daily requirements would be needed to support a weekly muscle mass gain of .5 to 1 kilograms (1 to 2 pounds) in addition to the energy requirements of the training (Reimers 2008).

To accomplish increased caloric intake, athletes should eat a larger amount of food just after the training session and smaller amounts before longer periods of rest (sleeping; Naclerio and Figueroa Alchapar 2011).

Conclusion

The daily energy requirement is determined by the sum of resting metabolic rate (RMR), thermic effect of food and the physical activity level. Several direct and indirect methods for estimating energy needs exist. Equations such as the Harris–Benedict formula along with other reference factors allow for an acceptable estimate of daily energy expenditure. Very restrictive or popular fad diets are not generally supported by science. Therefore even if some of their guidelines could be applied in some special cases, we do not recommend that these diets be included in healthy eating programmes. The optimal diet depends on many individual factors (e.g., age, sex, level of physical activities). In order to help athletes or special populations such as obese people achieve a well-balanced diet, personal trainers should use an individualised approach. To lose or gain weight, a low rate of decrease (1% of body weight per week) or increase (.5 to 1 kg maximum per week) is the accepted strategy for achieving an appropriate, healthy and stable outcome.

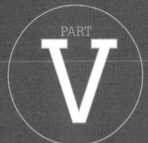

Training Adaptations, Exercise Planning and Programming ⇨⇨

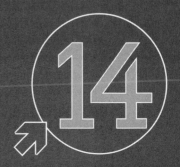

Training Adaptations

Rafael Oliveira

João Brito

Ben Jones

This chapter addresses several adaptations that occur in the body in response to a punctual stimulus or the training process. It should be read in conjunction with chapters 6 through 9 and 12 in *EuropeActive's Foundations for Exercise Professionals*. To achieve certain adjustments, clients must go through a training process; otherwise the body works to ensure *homeostasis*, or the constancy of the internal environment. The training process creates different conditions in the body through exercise adaptations in order to define a new state of balance. These adaptations are responses to stimuli or training processes that can have an acute or chronic character. The first stimulus (acute) refers to all the functional modifications that occur after the completion of the exercise. These may be sudden and temporary, disappearing shortly after the exercise (e.g., increased heart rate). The second stimulus (chronic) refers to a change that is more or less persistent in structure or function that follows the period of training and that allows the body to respond more easily to subsequent episodes of exercise (Maughan 2009).

Chronic adaptations improve our ability to keep various internal balances as close as possible to that of the resting state during intense exercise and to restore them immediately after its completion. For adaptation or improvement of a client's functional capacity, the exercise stimulus must be neither too weak (these will not overload the body), nor too strong (exhausting the body); rather personal trainers must choose an appropriate stimulus and apply it at the right time in the training programme (Hurley 1994). The adaptations will be more effective if the application of practice respects certain principles or basic laws.

As noted previously any adapted biological system is in dynamic equilibrium or homeostasis. If an exercise stimulus interrupts this homeostasis, the body tends to build a new balance by increasing regenerative, adaptive processes in order to protect the structure from future stimuli or stress. All adaptations, whether morphological, neuromuscular, cardiopulmonary or metabolic, depend on the principles that govern the training programme (Westcott 1995).

Adaptations to Training Principles

Skilled personal trainers blend science and art to deliver optimal results for their clients. Therefore they must have a basic understanding of the principles of training on which all exercise programmes are built as well as knowledge of how the body adapts to those principles.

Progressive Overload

This concept is sometimes broken down into separate principles of overload and progression, although they are intrinsically linked. The word *overload* describes the need to provide a new stimulus in order to provoke an adaptation in the body. *Progression* refers to the need to provide further new stimuli to cause continued adaptation.

For example if a sedentary person takes a brisk walk for 20 minutes, this will cause a state of overload in their body and stress their systems. After the walk their body will recover from this stress, and adaptations will occur throughout their various systems. If this person continues to walk for the same amount of time at the same pace daily, after a week or so their body will no longer need to adapt because the stimulus will no longer stress them beyond their capacity. In order to see further adaptation and improve their fitness, this person must progress the stimulus by working harder, for longer or with shorter recovery between bouts, or by changing the mode of exercise. The personal trainer has a duty to systematically implement these prerequisites into the training programme to assure training adaptation.

Specificity

Also known as the *SAID principle*, an acronym for specific adaptation to imposed demand, this concept refers to the observation that applying the principle of progressive overload to a particular activity stimulates adaptation, enabling the client to carry out that activity more easily over time. Although the response to any activity will involve the whole body and its specific systems, this response does not necessarily lead to a significant improvement in other types of activities.

The original research by Magel and colleagues (1975) in this area compared the effect of a 12-week swimming programme on performance in standardised tests of treadmill running and swimming ability. Although they anticipated that central adaptations of the cardiorespiratory system in particular would lead to an improvement in running ability, this was not observed. Further research has demonstrated similar results; therefore although cross-training using different exercise modalities is prevalent for active recovery in athletes, the primary mode of exercise must be the one in which they want to improve their performance. From a different perspective if a client has a more general fitness goal, particularly if they are exercising for weight management, they may benefit from using a range of training modalities to stimulate a wider range of adaptations, prevent tedium and reduce the risk of overuse injury.

The concept of specificity can be taken further in relation to sport, where not only the general mode of training, but also the specific movement patterns, rate of force development profiles and proprioceptive demand become relevant. Consider the following simple example: The joint action and therefore muscles involved in performing a lat pull-down exercise are the same as those used when performing a pull-up; however training using a lat pull-down will do little to improve the number of pull-ups a client can perform.

Reversibility

This is commonly expressed as the 'use it or lose it' principle. The process of adaptation to a stimulus following exercise stress is seen in the supercompensation curve in figure 14.1. This illustration shows how the stress of exercise causes an initial decrease in performance over the hours following exercise as cellular reactions requiring energy continue to occur, reducing the potential for fatigued and damaged cells to do work.

The recovery process soon kicks into action, and the affected cells are repaired over a timescale of 24 to 48 hours, to a point where the capacity for work is equal to that of the pre-exercise state. If no further exercise is performed at this time, adaptations occur and lead to *supercompensation*, the ability to perform at a higher level than in the pre-exercise state. If the next exercise session coincides

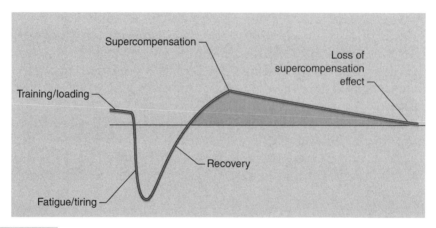

Figure 14.1 Supercompensation curve.

Reprinted, by permission, from V. Gambetta, 2007, *Athletic development: The art & science of functional sports conditioning* (Champaign, IL: Human Kinetics). 70.

at the peak of the supercompensation curve, and the exercise is progressed from the previous session to provide a suitable level of overload, the client will perform well and the recovery process will begin again from the new normal state.

If the client does not perform another exercise session during the period of supercompensation, the opportunity to progress is lost, and the adaptations from the initial exercise bout will revert to their pre-exercise state. Any further exercise sessions after this time will stimulate adaptation from the same starting point, and progression will be slow if it occurs at all. Among people who train consistently for a period of months or years, then stop exercising, the adaptations accumulated over time will gradually be lost. This detraining or reversibility is the adaptation of the body to the absence of a need to maintain the capacity for a level of work it is no longer required to perform.

Adaptability

Adaptability is not so much a principle of training as a principle for life. The ability to adapt plans on the spot in response to an unexpected change in the situation, but still use the client's time productively to work towards their goals is a skill worth developing for personal trainers. It is not uncommon for a client to arrive at a training session in an unfit state to complete the rigorous programme the personal trainer had planned because they had performed an impromptu exercise session the day before. In these cases the personal trainer must be able to think on the spot, determining which programme variables can be adapted to give the client a level of intensity and challenge that will be productive.

Individuality

Because personal training is commonly offered as a one-to-one approach, this principle is crucial. The principle of individuality or individual difference states that the response of any two people to the same training stimulus will be different. The introduction to this chapter emphasises the concept of personal training as the art of applying a scientific approach with the flexibility to respond to the needs of a client. This is a vital concept to grasp in order to succeed as a personal trainer. Human beings are not machines, and the client's exact response to an external stress such as exercise will inevitably retain a degree of unpredictability. Personal trainers must carefully observe their clients and make a conscious effort to acutely attend to their verbal and non-verbal feedback when performing exercises. The most carefully planned programme is irrelevant if the client is not ready to perform the planned session when they arrive on any given day.

Recovery Time

Recovery time is the amount of time required after an exercise session for the body to adapt adequately before performing another session. This programme variable is governed by the supercompensation curve of the individual client at any point in time. Guidelines for recovery time include allowing 24 to 72 hours of rest between intense exercise sessions of similar type. But these guidelines are just that. Some deconditioned and highly stressed clients with poor nutrient intake may have barely recovered enough to train again after 72 hours, whilst a highly conditioned athlete with optimal nutrition and nothing to focus on but eating, sleeping and training may be capable of performing intense sessions twice per day without detriment in the short term.

Adaptations to Resistance Training

The term *resistance training* immediately conjures an image of Olympic weightlifting for most people; however all forms of training that involve moving the body against an external force can be considered resistance training. When defined in this way any movement that requires the body to produce force in order to overcome a force outside of the body is a resistance training exercise. The key variable of resistance training is the amount of force that the body needs to generate in response to the forces it must overcome. The muscular fitness continuum in figure 14.2 is a useful tool for visualising this concept.

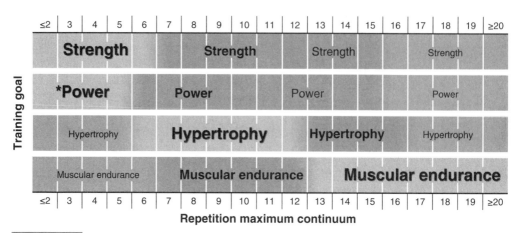

≤2	3	4	5	6	7	8	9	10	11	12	13	14	15	16	17	18	19	≥20

Figure 14.2   The muscular fitness continuum.

Reprinted, by permission, from NSCA, 2008, Resistance training, by T.R. Baechle, R.W. Earle, and D. Wathen. In *Essentials of strength training and conditioning,* 3rd ed., edited by T.R. Baechle and R.W. Earle (Champaign, IL: Human Kinetics), 401.

Neuromuscular Adaptations

The size principle of motor unit recruitment describes the pattern in which motor units, and therefore muscle fibres, are recruited. The brain will activate only the minimum number of motor units required to perform a task. To make movement as efficient as possible, the first motor units to be recruited are the smallest ones within that muscle. These small motor units innervate Type I (slow oxidative) muscle fibres. As greater forces are required, or when these motor units begin to fatigue, larger motor units innervating Type IIa (fast oxidative glycolytic) muscle fibres will be recruited. In order to generate high levels of force or create explosive movement, the largest motor units innervating the Type IIx (fast glycolytic) muscle fibres will be recruited. Figure 14.3 shows the relationship between force production and muscle fibre recruitment. Each motor unit will innervate only muscle fibres of a homogenous type (Reilly et al. 1990).

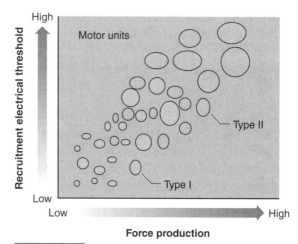

Figure 14.3   Size principle of motor unit recruitment.

Reprinted, by permission, from NSCA, 2008, Adaptations to anaerobic training programs, by N.A. Ratamess. In *Essentials of strength training and conditioning,* 3rd ed., edited by T.R. Baechle and R.W. Earle (Champaign, IL: Human Kinetics), 97.

The muscle growth that results from resistance training is called *hypertrophy*. It is the result of increasing the cross-sectional area of muscle fibres. The process of hypertrophy involves an increase in the synthesis of the proteins myosin and actin (primary components of myofilaments) and also an increase in the number of myofibrils of the muscle fibre (Maughan 2009). Hypertrophy does not occur uniformly in the various types of muscle fibres. Several studies have found that the fast-twitch fibres (Type II) have an increase greater than the slow-twitch fibres (Type I). In fact the client's potential for hypertrophy involves their proportion of fast fibres in relation to slow fibres (Maughan 2009). The differences in the composition of the muscle fibres and their number partially explain the variability among different people in hypertrophic responses to training. The kind of training also influences different adaptations of muscle fibres (Maughan 2009).

Hypertrophic responses are influenced by the client's training history. Among sedentary people increases in strength during the first and second months of training are not usually accompanied by a significant hypertrophy of muscle fibres. Strength gains in this initial period of training are thought to be derived from the adjustments of the neural factors (Maughan 2009).

According to some studies, a month of detraining results in a negligible loss of strength and muscle cross-section. After this period the reduction in strength occurs faster than the decrease of muscle fibres. This fact suggests that the loss of neural adaptations is the main reason for the decrease in strength after 2 to 3 months of detraining.

Adaptations to Specific Programmes

The principle of specificity states that the type of resistance training programme dictates the specific changes or adaptations that occur in the body. The primary goals of resistance training are maximum strength, hypertrophy, power and muscular endurance (Baechle and Earle 2008).

A resistance training programme designed to maximise strength is characterised by high loads and low number of repetitions (1 to 6 repetitions). This kind of training causes greater hypertrophy of Type II fibres relative to Type I. Type II fibres produce higher levels of strength and speed than Type I. The muscle adapts biochemically to this type of training, increasing the reserves of energy substrates such as muscle glycogen, creatine phosphate and adenosine triphosphate (ATP). The amount and the activity of glycolytic enzymes and enzymes that renew adenosine triphosphate also increase with training (Maughan 2009).

A resistance training programme designed to increase muscle size involves moderate loads that allow clients to perform 6 to 12 repetitions until fatigue. The rest interval time is shorter so that clients can complete the next series before the full recovery. Biochemical adaptations are similar to those that occur with strength training, although the increased levels of creatine phosphate have a greater influence on the client's ability to develop strength after 20 to 30 seconds of exercise; this is important because each series lasts an average of 30 to 90 seconds (Maughan 2009).

A resistance training programme that uses submaximal muscle contractions over a long period of time with numerous repetitions (12 to 25 maximum repetitions) with reduced rest periods will improve muscular endurance. This type of training increases the oxidative potential of Type I and Type IIa fibres, as well as oxidative enzyme activity (Krebs cycle). At the cellular level there is an increase in the number and size of the mitochondria, which are responsible for ATP production via aerobic oxidation of glycogen (Westcott 1986).

Specific adaptations to high-intensity, low-volume resistance training for strength include the following:

- Increased maximal strength
- Greater recruitment and rate of discharge of motor units
- Increased muscle cross-sectional area
- Changes in muscle architecture
- Possible adaptations to increased metabolites (e.g., H^+)

Specific adaptations to low-intensity, high-volume resistance training for muscular endurance include the following:

- Improved absolute and relative local muscle endurance
- Increased mitochondrial size and number
- Increased glycogen storage capacity
- Selective increase in cross-sectional diameter of Type I and Type IIa fibres
- Increase in capillary density

Resistance training programmes can be progressed in a wide variety of ways, not least through using different means of loading (e.g., barbell, dumbbell, cable, elastic resistance) to give a different force profile and stimulus to the body. Variations of exercise technique that place stress on different areas and challenge co-ordination through unfamiliar or complex movement patterns will also progress a training programme, and they can make traditional exercises more relevant to sport or everyday life. The main variables manipulated in resistance training programmes, however, are volume and intensity. The same exercise routine performed using loads at different ends of the muscular fitness continuum leads to very different adaptations, and training between these extremes produces a mixture of these adaptations.

Bone Adaptations

Even though bone is a rigid structure, it is actually a very active tissue. When subjected to forces bone has the capacity for growth and regeneration. Exercise provides forces that can cause tension in specific regions of the skeleton. These include twisting, bending and compression forces created by the muscle contractions at the muscle's tendon insertion on the bone. In response to mechanical forces, bone cells called *osteoblasts* migrate to the surface of the bone suffering from the tension for the process of *bone remodelling*. Osteoblasts produce proteins, the molecules of collagen, which settle in the spaces between the bone cells in order to increase the strength of the bone in that area. These proteins form the bone matrix. The matrix proteins mineralise into calcium phosphate crystals. This protein mineralisation gives bone its rigidity (Maughan 2009). Bone formation occurs predominantly at its surface, called the *periosteum*.

Bone growth is similar to muscle growth in response to exercise. The adaptation of bone to mechanical forces occurs at different levels, as in the case of axial bone (spine and proximal part of femur) or the appendicular skeleton (long bones). The growth of trabecular bone tissue (spongy) is different from that of cortical bone tissue (compact). Trabecular bone responds more quickly to stimuli than does cortical bone. The loss of the bone matrix and bone mineral density after a period of stimulation or reduction of immobility occurs faster than the formation and bone mineralisation (Maughan 2009).

Adaptations to Aerobic Training

Adaptations to aerobic (also referred to as *cardiorespiratory*) training are primarily due to changes in the heart, lungs and vascular system.

Cardiovascular Adaptations

Aerobic endurance depends on the ability of the body to carry oxygen to the tissues to satisfy their energy needs. For this process to be effective the body must have a good ability to capture, secure, transport and use oxygen (O_2). This efficiency is expressed in terms of the consumption of O_2 per minute ($\dot{V}O_2$). The cardiovascular system plays an important role during aerobic exercise because it is responsible for transporting nutrients and metabolites resulting from metabolic processes, removing carbon dioxide, maintaining body temperature and controlling pH (ACSM 2012).

The heart increases its weight and volume with this kind of training, which aims to improve the heart's ability to withstand moderate efforts over a long period of time. This increase occurs primarily in the left ventricular cavity, which contracts more powerfully as a result of the training (ACSM 2012; Maughan 2009).

At rest, the average heart rate is 60 to 90 beats per minute, but sedentary people can have values close to 100 beats per minute. Well-trained aerobic endurance athletes can have resting heart rate values between 28 and 40 beats per minute. Resting heart rate varies with age and with environmental changes such as temperature and altitude (ACSM 2012). During exercise heart rate increases rapidly, and heart rate is directly proportional to the intensity of exercise. Maximum heart rate is calculated with the client's age; from year to year maximum heart rate shows a reduction of a beat per minute (Gellish et al. 2007).

In relation to *cardiac output* (heart rate times stroke volume), there are no differences between trained and untrained clients at rest. During submaximal aerobic exercise, trained clients will have a slight decrease compared to untrained clients. During maximal exercise, however, trained clients will have a greater cardiac output compared to untrained clients because of their larger heart volume and capacity for a higher maximal heart rate (Baechle and Earle 2008).

As clients adapt to anaerobic exercise, they experience an increase of the anaerobic threshold. This change occurs due to the body's increased capacity to remove the lactic acid produced and an increase of enzyme concentration and enzyme activities (Brooks 1986).

Systolic blood pressure increases in proportion with the intensity of the exercise. During exercise diastolic pressure values have smaller amplitudes of change than those of systolic blood pressure (increases of only about 15 mmHg compared to about 50 mmHg; Westcott 1993). Due to training adaptations resting blood pressure has a tendency to decrease in clients with elevated blood pressure (hypertension); systolic blood pressure may lower about 11 mmHg and diastolic blood pressure may lower about 8 mmHg (Westcott 1993).

Respiratory Adaptations

During aerobic exercise, many changes in the acid–base balance (pH) are caused by the difference between oxygen and carbon dioxide in the blood. These are quantified through the respiratory exchange ratio (RER). A way of controlling the pH is through breathing. The increase in ventilation occurs as a response to mechanical motion and the physiological response related to the increased need to expel CO_2. This consequently lowers pH levels by stimulating the chemo-receptors and increasing ventilation. Thus two phases can be distinguished: a mechanical phase and a physiological phase resulting from increases in temperature, pH and blood pressure (ACSM 2012; Maughan 2009).

Increases in ventilation are also due to increased *tidal volume* (mobilised air between the beginning and the end of a normal inspiration). During more intense exercise this increase is mainly due to increased respiratory frequency. The *pulmonary diffusion*, which is the exchange of gases (O_2 and CO_2) that occurs in the alveoli, remains unchanged at rest or after a submaximal exercise. However it increases during maximum exercise in which there is a greater flow of blood to the lung region and higher pulmonary diffusion (ACSM 2012; Maughan 2009).

The difference between the percentage of O_2 in arterial and venous blood increases with practice. Adaptations to aerobic training improve the ability to exercise at a given oxygen consumption (i.e., intensity level) without increasing blood lactate concentration levels (ACSM 2012; Maughan 2009). Maximal oxygen consumption ($\dot{V}O_2$max) can increase as much as 20 percent in sedentary people after 3 to 6 months of following an aerobic training programme that involves an intensity of 75 percent of $\dot{V}O_2$max (Hurley et al. 1988).

Adaptations to Range of Motion Training

Range of motion (ROM) training is commonly referred to as *stretching*. The main types of stretching are static (which can be further subdivided into *active* and *passive*), dynamic range of movement, ballistic and proprioceptive neuromuscular facilitation (PNF), which can be further subdivided into *contract-relax* and *contract-relax-agonist-contract* protocols.

Adaptations to Specific Techniques

The principle of specificity states that the type of stretching technique used dictates the specific changes or adaptations that occur in the body.

Static stretching is the most commonly accepted and practised method of improving flexibility. It has been shown to be effective at increasing range of movement. Although this is rarely disputed, other adaptations that are less supported by the literature include relief of delayed-onset muscle soreness, enhanced athletic performance and reduced injury risk. The main concerns about static stretching are the downregulation of the protective stretch reflex and the poor correlation of static flexibility to active range of movement. Static stretching increases the difference between the zones of active and passive inadequacy around a joint and therefore may promote injury risk (ACSM 2013).

Dynamic ROM stretching is sometimes considered under the banner of ballistic stretching, with the key difference being the smooth speed of movement within the client's current ROM. This is in contrast to the generally faster and more forceful ballistic stretching, which aims to force the joint past its current range. Dynamic ROM stretching is not often used as a means of improving ROM long term, but it is commonly used as a means of preparation for unloaded movement as part of a warm-up routine.

Ballistic stretching has been demonstrated to be effective at improving ROM in a similar magnitude to static stretching. The main arguments against this method of stretching are that inadequate time is given for tissue adaptation, soreness results from injury to soft tissues, the stretch reflex is initiated and neurological adaptation may be inadequate (ACSM 2013). Conversely the major argument for ballistic stretching is the development of dynamic flexibility. The general population should avoid ballistic stretching. When introduced with an athletic population, it should be done progressively.

Personal trainers often employ PNF stretching in the fitness setting because it provides an opportunity for client interaction and a more impressive immediate flexibility improvement than static stretching does, although the long-term increase in ROM is comparable to that achieved with static stretching (ACSM 2007).

Conclusion

Exercise performed as part of an overall training programme induces profound acute and chronic adaptations in the structure and function of the musculoskeletal and cardiovascular systems. Training adaptations are specific to the type of programme followed and the manipulation of the principles that comprise the specific training programme. A summary of the primary adaptations is seen in table 14.1.

This chapter explains the main neuromuscular, bone, cardiovascular and respiratory adaptations that occur with exercise training. Personal trainers need this knowledge for safe and effective exercise planning and programming that is based on the client's goals (see chapter 15).

Table 14.1 Adaptations to Resistance, Cardiovascular and ROM Training

Variable	Observed with resistance training	Observed with cardiovascular training	Observed with ROM training
Cardiovascular system			
Myocardial mass	↑	↑↑↑	↔
Stroke volume	↑	↑↑↑	↔
Resting heart rate	↓	↓↓↓	↔
Resting blood pressure	↓↓	↓↓↓	↔
Capillary density	↑ from low load, high repetitions ↓ from high load, low repetitions	↑↑↑	↔
Blood volume	?	↑↑↑	↔
Erythrocyte quantity	?	↑↑↑	↔
Skeletal system			
Bone mass and bone mineral density	↑ from adequate loads (>10RM)	↑ from impact loading activities only (e.g., running)	↔
Joint ROM	↑ from full ROM movements only	↔ or ↓ (activity and volume dependent)	↑↑↑
Muscular system			
Fibre cross-sectional area	↑ to ↑↑↑ (depending on the training protocol)	↓	↔
Muscle mass	↓ to ↑↑↑ (depending on the training protocol)	↓	↔
Mitochondrial size and density	↑↑ to ↔ (depending on the training protocol)	↑↑↑	↔
Nervous system			
Motor unit recruitment	↑↑↑ but specific to load, movements and velocities used	↑ but specific to mode of training used	↔ or ↓
Synchronisation of motor unit activation	↑ from low to moderate loads ↑↑↑ from heavy, explosive lifting	↑ but specific to mode of training used	↔

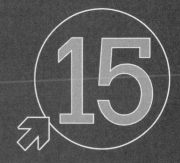

Exercise Planning and Programming

Christoffer Andersen

Thomas Rieger

Lars L. Andersen

Against the background of EuropeActive's main vision of getting more people to be more active, the majority of personal trainer courses and related learning outcomes in Europe are aimed at the health-oriented client who seeks to feel healthier, look better or lose body weight. Therefore exercise planning and programming primarily considers the aforementioned target group as having the highest relevance.

This chapter on standards in fitness represents a useful and easy-to-understand addition to other chapters in the EuropeActive book series. Readers should familiarise themselves with the content of the following chapters of *EuropeActive's Foundations for Exercise Professionals*: Components and Principles of Fitness (chapter 6), Resistance Training (chapter 7), Aerobic Training (chapter 8), Flexibility Training (chapter 9) and Progression (chapter 12). Readers should also consult these chapters from *EuropeActive's Essentials for Fitness Instructors*: Cardiorespiratory Exercise (chapter 3), Resistance Exercise (chapter 4), Safe Progressive Exercise Planning (chapter 5) and Preparing Fitness Programmes (chapter 6). Based on the learning outcomes from these chapters, the main purpose of this one is to emphasise selected information with regard to the special requirements of exercise planning and programming. The most obvious characteristic of personal training is the one-to-one approach. The specifics of this approach are applied to the planning and programming processes for the most crucial types of exercise, resistance and aerobic endurance training. Finally integrated exercise programmes for different cases are provided.

Planning for Resistance Training

Among the other fitness components, strength plays a key role in helping clients achieve their fitness-related goals. New research studies have shown how important muscle mass is in terms of overall health, metabolic efficiency and disease prevention (Pedersen 2011; Pedersen and Hojman 2012). Due to the steadily increasing importance of muscle strength and muscle mass related to different health indicators, resistance training is pivotal in personal training programmes. To get the whole picture of resistance training, read this section in conjunction with chapter 7 in *EuropeActive's Foundations for Exercise Professionals* and chapter 4 in *EuropeActive's Essentials for Fitness Instructors*.

Progressive Overload

Resistance training programmes increase or maintain strength or muscle mass. To attain results beyond our current physical capacity, our muscles need to be challenged with heavier loads or more repetitions. This challenge stimulates the adaptive processes of the muscular and nervous systems, forcing the body to cope with the new demands placed on it. Progressive overload is the gradual increase of stress placed on the muscles during resistance training (e.g., by lifting heavier weights or attempting to squeeze out another repetition). The system of progressive overload is often attributed to Captain Thomas Delorme, MD, who systematically used this approach to rehabilitate soldiers after the Second World War (Delorme and Watkins 1948). Progressive overload is a fundamental principle for success in various forms of training programmes, including fitness training, weightlifting, high-intensity training and physical therapy. Progressive overload is crucial for continuously stimulating muscle growth and strengthening the skeletal system (Fleck and Kraemer 2014; Kraemer and Fleck 2007; Ratamess et al. 2009). Furthermore progressive overload stimulates the development of the nervous system, resulting in more efficient and stronger nerve impulses to the muscles and, consequently, stronger and more powerful muscles. Personal trainers should be very accurate about their client's progress, which shows the steps made towards the overall goal of the training period. Personal trainers must thoroughly document each workout in terms of volume and intensity, and should always try to help their clients progress in small increments. This is what professional planning in resistance training is all about, defining sub-goals in advance, documenting them and afterwards explaining to the client how successful the training period was. From a psychological standpoint this explanation is very important because experiencing success helps clients stay on track.

Specificity

Training adaptations are specific to the stimulus applied. Consequently resistance training programmes should be designed to meet the client's specific goal. The factors that determine the physiological adaptations to resistance training include muscle groups, speed of muscle contraction, range of motion, muscle actions, repetitions, intensity, volume and frequency of training (Siff 2003; Fleck and Kramer 2014; Zatsiorsky and Kraemer 2006).

Progression in resistance training means moving forwards or working towards a specific goal within a defined time frame until the target goal has been achieved. To achieve a specific goal through resistance training, personal trainers should consider the aforementioned factors, not just choosing the right exercise for the right muscle. The adaptations following resistance training are specific to the intensity with which the exercises were performed. Table 15.1 shows basic recommendations for intermediate trainees for different training goals.

As seen in the preceding table strength primarily comes from training with a high intensity. At this intensity, it is possible to perform only a few repetitions because the fastest motor units fatigue rapidly. This causes limited fatigue in the involved muscles. The adaptations are therefore to a large extent neural, although hypertrophy of large fast-twitch muscle fibres also occurs. In personal training, where health-oriented clients, beginners or intermediate trainees are primarily addressed, the high-intensity training in between 90 and 100 percent of maximum effort can be neglected, because the application of heavy resistance makes the risk of injuries very high.

At the other end of the scale is muscular endurance, which comes from performing many repetitions with a relatively low intensity. During these longer-lasting sets metabolites build up in the muscles involved, and the predominant adaptations are enzymatic within the trained muscles. The main hypertrophy range requires activation of almost all motor units and buildup of significant fatigue within the muscle. Exhausting the muscles with several sets of fairly heavy loads is considered a bulletproof recipe for attaining muscle mass.

Table 15.1 Resistance Training Guidelines for Different Training Goals

| | Training goal | | | |
Variable	Strength	Power	Hypertrophy	Muscular endurance
Load (% of 1RM)	80-90	45-55	60-80	40-60
Repetitions per set	1-5	1-5	6-12	15-60
Sets per exercise	4-7	3-5	4-8	2-4
Rest between sets (minutes)	2-6	2-6	2-5	1-2
Duration (seconds per set)	5-10	4-8	20-60	80-150
Speed per repetition (% of max)	60-100	90-100	60-90	60-80
Training sessions per week	3-6	3-6	5-7	8-14

Note that other sources provide guidelines slightly different than what is provided here. See chapter 7 in *EuropeActive's Foundations for Exercise Professionals* and chapter 4 in *EuropeActive's Essentials for Fitness Instructors* for more information.

Reprinted, by permission, from M.C. Siff, 2003, *Supertraining,* 6th ed. (Denver, CO: Supertraining Institute).

Hypertrophy can also be obtained with fewer repetitions if the total volume is high (i.e., requiring many sets). Recent studies have also found some evidence of hypertrophy in response to high-repetition resistance training consisting of more than 20 consecutive repetitions to failure.

However, when working with untrained clients, multiple-set resistance training offers only small benefits over single-set training with respect to either strength gain or muscle mass increase, but for the well-trained client, multiple-set systems are required for optimal progress (Ratamess et al. 2009). Strength adaptations during the initial months of strength training occur largely through adaptations of the nervous system, both in terms of gross motor learning as well as increased neuronal firing of specific motor units. This should be taken into consideration in developing exercise programmes for the aforementioned client group. A certain volume of training is desirable in untrained clients to attain these adaptations fast. Therefore personal trainers should begin clients with sets of 10 to 15 repetitions, using strict form with loading; clients could perform these for 20 repetitions if only one set to failure were performed. For the untrained client, optimal training frequency is approximately three times per week. For the more well-trained client, the largest gains are seen with slightly higher intensity—around 6RM on average—and a training frequency of only two times per week for each muscle group (Fleck and Kraemer 2014; Ratamess et al. 2009). Note that the result will be more total training sessions per week (i.e., 4 or 5 depending on how the 2 sessions per muscle group are spread out throughout the week).

Exercise Order

Personal trainers should always be aware that the exercise programme must be derived from the desired adaptations. This also applies when exercises are sequenced based on relationships between agonist and antagonist muscle groups. Muscle force and power may be increased when antagonist movements are performed; however force and power may be reduced if the exercises are performed consecutively. Performance of compound exercises (e.g., bench press, squats in different variations, leg press, and shoulder press) declines significantly when these exercises are performed later (after several exercises stressing similar muscle groups) rather than earlier in a workout. Considering that these compound exercises are effective for increasing strength and hypertrophy, maximising performance of these exercises by performing them early in a workout may be necessary for optimal strength gains (Fleck and Kraemer 2014; Ratamess et al. 2009; Siff 2003; Zatsiorsky and Kraemer 2006).

The basic rules for exercise order are to place the following types first in the training session:

- Compound exercises with high demands for the nervous system
- High-intensity exercises with high loads and few repetitions
- Goal-specific exercises

The following can be performed later in the training session:

- Single-joint exercises
- Fatiguing exercises with medium load and several repetitions
- Exercises for the stabilising musculature
- Assistive exercises

In this regard the relation of supervised and unsupervised sessions comes into play. Due to the complexity of the compound movements personal trainers should try to plan sessions with supervision in a training cycle, when these sessions are strength-training dominant.

To help their clients avoid bad posture and other problematic movement patterns, personal trainers can develop cues and commands.

Advanced Techniques

Several techniques are used to challenge the muscles to adapt beyond their current capability. Bodybuilders and recreational athletes have used many of the techniques in this section for decades. Many clients use these techniques to force themselves past a plateau. Nevertheless be aware that these techniques are to be used only for motivated clients, since they are as exhausting as they are effective (Fleck and Kraemer 2014; Siff 2003). Personal trainers must not overstrain their clients with these advanced techniques. An appropriate balance between high-intensity elements that likely lead to the wanted adaptations and phases of moderate intensity is key to keeping clients motivated, minimising the likelihood they will drop out and helping them achieve their training goals.

Drop Sets

Drop sets do not end at the point of momentary muscular failure, but continue with progressively lighter weights. For example, when failure is reached during the first set, the client should immediately drop 30 percent of the load and continue to failure with the lighter set.

Pyramid Sets

In pyramid sets the progression is from lighter weights with a greater number of repetitions in the first set, to heavier weights with fewer repetitions in subsequent sets. Pyramid sets have been criticised for fatiguing the muscles before the really heavy and effective sets are performed. Therefore the reverse pyramid has gained popularity. A reverse pyramid follows the opposite pattern: heavier weights are used at the beginning, and then the load is progressively lightened.

Supersets

Supersets combine two or more exercises to maximise the amount of work done in a certain amount of time. The exercises are performed with minimal or no rest period between them.

Antagonistic Supersets

Antagonistic supersets are similar to regular supersets, but they involve exercises that work opposing muscle groups (e.g., during arm exercises, combining biceps curls with the triceps push-down). Other examples include the military press and pull-down and the bench press and wide grip row combinations. This way the prime movers from one exercise recover whilst the antagonistic muscles work in the second exercise.

Pre- and Postexhaustion

Pre-exhaustion combines an isolation exercise with a compound exercise for the same muscle group. The isolation exercise first exhausts the muscle group, and then the compound exercise uses the supporting muscles to push the initial group further than would otherwise be possible. A popular combination is the dumbbell chest fly combined with the bench press. For many clients the triceps fatigue quickly during the bench press, thereby limiting the stimulus on the pectoral muscles. However by pre-exhausting the pectoral muscles using the dumbbell chest fly exercise, the pectorals and triceps will fail simultaneously during the subsequent bench press, and both will benefit equally from the exercise. This approach can also be used in corrective exercise therapy if a client has gluteal amnesia: The client can perform supine hip thrusts as an isolation exercise to activate and fatigue the gluteal muscles before performing squats or lunges as compound exercises. When the compound exercise is done first followed by the isolation exercise, it is called *postexhaustion*. This is used to exhaust weak or lagging muscles even further; the load used in the compound exercise will not be compromised by fatigue from the isolation exercise.

Breakdowns

Breakdowns work the different types of muscle fibres for maximum stimulation. Three different exercises that work the same muscle group are selected and then used as a superset. The first exercise uses a heavy weight (~85 percent of one-repetition max, or 1RM) for around 5 repetitions, the second a medium weight (~70 percent of 1RM) for around 12 repetitions, and finally the third exercise uses a light weight (~50 percent of 1RM) for 20 to 30 repetitions, or even lighter (~40 percent of 1RM) for 40 or more repetitions. Going to failure is discouraged.

Forced Repetitions

Forced repetitions occur after momentary muscular failure. A spotter provides just enough help to get the client past the sticking point of the exercise and complete further repetitions. Clients often do this when they are spotting their exercise partner. With some exercises forced repetitions can be done without a spotter. For example with one-arm biceps curls, the other arm can be used to assist the arm that is being trained.

Rest-Pause (Post-Failure)

After a normal set of 6 to 8 repetitions (to failure), the client racks the weight for 15 to 30 seconds and then performs a couple more repetitions. This process can be repeated for two or three more sets with a few repetitions. The 20-repetition breathing squats is a similar approach in that it follows a 10RM set of squats with individual rest-pause repetitions, up to a total of 20 repetitions.

Negative Repetitions (Eccentrics)

Negative repetitions are performed with much heavier weights. A spotter lifts the weight, and then the client lowers it in a controlled manner through an eccentric contraction. Alternatively a client can use an exercise machine for negatives by lifting the weight with both arms or legs and then lowering it with only one. Or they can simply lower weights more slowly than they lift them, for example, by taking 2 seconds to lift each weight and 4 seconds to lower it.

Partial Repetitions

Partial repetitions, as the name implies, involve movement through only part of the normal path of an exercise. Partial repetitions can be performed with very heavy weights that could not be lifted even once during a full range of motion. Usually only the easiest part of the repetition is attempted (e.g., squats in a safety rack bending only slightly [30 degrees] in the knees). Unless there is a specific functional purpose, full range of motion is normally advised for optimal strength and hypertrophy in spite of the lower loads used.

Rest-Pause (Heavy Singles)

Rest-pause heavy singles are performed near 1RM, with 10 to 20 seconds of rest between each repetition, and are repeated six to eight times. Personal trainers should use this method infrequently.

Calculating Resistance Training Intensity

The number of repetitions a person can perform at a certain weight is called the *repetition maximum* (RM). For example, if a client can perform 10 repetitions with 75 kilograms, then in the specific exercise their RM for that weight would be 10RM. 1RM is therefore the maximum weight that someone can lift in a given exercise (i.e., the weight that they can lift only once without a break), and it is equal to 100 percent intensity for that exercise. Instead of using a percentage of maximum it is more practical to use the RM measurement because there is a direct correlation between the two. 1RM can also be used as an upper limit in order to determine the desired load for an exercise (as a percentage of the 1RM).

As seen in table 15.1, various resistance training goals call for lifting a certain percentage of the client's 1RM. However many consider the risk of injury when attempting a 1RM to be higher than when performing multiple repetition sets. Therefore there have been various proposals for ways to calculate an approximation of the 1RM. Two common formulas used to calculate IRM follow (r is the number of repetitions performed and w is the amount of weight used).

Formula 1

$$1RM = [r/30 + 1] \times w$$

Formula 2

This version of the 1RM calculation is often called the Brzycki formula. It can be written either in terms of integers or decimal approximation (Brzycki 1998):

$$1RM = w \times 36/(37 - r)$$
$$= w/[37/36 - (1/36 \times r)]$$
$$\approx w/[1.0278 - (0.0278 \times r)]$$

Formulas 1 and 2 return identical results for 10 repetitions. However for fewer than 10 repetitions, formula 1 returns a slightly higher estimated maximum. For example if a person can lift 100 kilograms on a given exercise for 10 repetitions, the estimated 1RM would be 133 kilograms for both formulas. However if the person were to complete only 6 repetitions, then formula 1 would estimate a 1RM of approximately 120 kilograms and formula 2 would return an estimate of approximately 116 kilograms. These types of calculations may not always produce accurate results, but they can be used as starting points. The weight can then be changed in practice as needed to perform the number of repetitions called for by the training programme. Calculators using submaximal loads are also used to predict 1RM. The degree of accuracy can vary greatly depending on the exercise and the client's weight training experience and muscular composition.

Mobility

Particularly when training compound movements like squats, dead lifts or any kind of overhead movements, resistance training sessions must regularly be complemented by related mobility work for the involved joints (Starrett and Cordoza 2013).

Planning for Aerobic Endurance Training

Due to its importance alongside resistance training, aerobic endurance activity should be considered against the specific conditions of personal training. Chapter 3 in *EuropeActive's Essentials for Fitness Instructors* (Benvenuti and Zanuso 2015) and chapter 7 of this book build the substantial basis for the following paragraphs.

General Factors

Aerobic endurance training encompasses different modes of activities that primarily stress the aerobic energy system and produce a number of cardiovascular and respiratory adaptations that increase aerobic endurance (ACSM 2011). High levels of aerobic fitness are obligatory not only for high performance athletes but also for regular clients who want to improve their overall fitness. Personal trainers must know that aerobic endurance training programmes should mirror the one taking place for resistance training. They must also decide about types of exercise, exercise order, intensity, volume, rest intervals (if interval training is preferred), frequency and so forth.

How these parameters are arranged depends on the client's goal. As mentioned before goal achievement is always pivotal. Clients will never rehire a personal trainer if they do not reach their determined goals. Personal training is similar to all other businesses: If their expectations are not satisfied, clients will seek other options. Thus it is crucial that the goal-setting process in aerobic endurance training is as precise as possible. In this regard the mode of aerobic endurance training is very important. If the personal trainer is supervising the aerobic endurance training session (for a better understanding of the relation between supervised and unsupervised sessions, see chapter 2), they should choose a mode that allows them to monitor the client's heart rate so that they can intervene easily (e.g., every indoor activity on an ergometer, jogging or walking outdoors). According to the primary target group for personal training, namely the novice or average person, goals like improvement of stamina and fat loss are more important than extreme performance enhancement for elite athletes. The latter should be discussed in following publications representing other educational standards.

Calculating Aerobic Training Intensity

To improve a client's aerobic capacity, the personal trainer has to determine a client's training intensity. Based on the client's fitness level, the personal trainer calculates their exercise heart rate as being within a low-, medium- or high-intensity training zone.

For the untrained client, there are several ways to improve stamina through aerobic endurance training. The first one is the low-intensity steady state (LISS) method, which is performed with a heart rate between 50 and 65 percent of the maximum heart rate (HRmax) for a duration of 30 to 60 minutes, depending on the client's fitness status. For this method the increase of duration must be applied first. The second possibility is more interval oriented. The most popular routines in this regard are Fartlek training and high-intensity interval training (HIIT). Both approaches are characterised by sequences of high intensity and a heart rate between 70 and 80 percent of HRmax, interrupted by rest intervals aiming to decrease heart rate to the low-intensity training zone within a time frame of 30 to 60 seconds. How do these different methods affect the planning process of personal training? It again depends on the relationship between supervised and unsupervised sessions. If the personal trainer decides that the best method for the client is the LISS approach, they should plan the majority of sessions to be unsupervised because it is quite easy for clients to monitor intensity on their own. Thus the personal trainer can invest more time in the support of the resistance training. If the choice is interval training, the situation is different. Supervision is important because intensity changes periodically and heart rate monitoring gets more challenging. In addition the client may be inexperienced at interval training.

Applied Training Programming

In terms of programming, success depends on the optimal balance between load and recovery. Hence the supercompensation theory explained in chapter 14 is relevant for all types of training. Additionally periodisation is a key applied programming strategy, not only to assure training success, but also to avoid boredom and keep motivation levels high.

Application of the Supercompensation Theory

Although the supercompensation theory applies to resistance training as well as aerobic endurance training, a common application is a resistance training program designed to improve muscular strength.

A client begins a resistance training session with a certain level of muscular strength. As the training session progresses, their level of strength decreases due to fatigue (i.e., the client cannot perform as many repetitions with the same weight, or their ability to lift a certain amount of weight decreases). In the time period after the training session, the client's body gradually recovers and the strength level increases up to the initial strength level. Then, due to the body's ability to adapt to imposed demands, strength will increase beyond the initial baseline. In other words the increase in strength following a training session does not stop at the initial strength level; rather it enters a period of supercompensation during which strength surpasses the initial level. However if the client completes no further workouts or goes for a longer time without training, their strength level will gradually decrease back towards the initial level. If subsequent workouts take place too soon, no progress will occur, possibly leading to a vicious circle resulting in overtraining. If the next workout takes place during the supercompensation period, the body will advance to a higher level of fitness. If the next workout takes place after the supercompensation period, the body will remain at the base level.

In the more advanced levels of training, some workouts are intentionally scheduled during the recovery period; these are followed by a longer rest period to achieve greater supercompensation effects (Fleck and Kraemer 2014; Kraemer and Fleck 2007; Zatsiorsky and Kraemer 2006).

Relationship Between Supercompensation and Training Programmes

With the supercompensation theory in mind, creating effective training programs appears simple. A personal trainer needs to know only how much the training taps into the initial fitness and how much recovery is needed for supercompensation. Afterwards training continues at the same intensity level, with necessary intervals between workouts required for supercompensation. However the muscular and nervous systems are made up of numerous tissues, which all have different optimal supercompensation times (Zatsiorsky and Kraemer 2006).

Further recovery speed for each tissue is affected by training intensity and volume, nutrition, stress, sleep and other variables. To make it even more complex the aforementioned functions and parameters are basic ones. Muscle strength and mass are complex parameters. Muscle mass is a function of many different simple parameters. For example the amount of glycogen in muscles is a basic parameter that influences muscle mass. The basic guidelines are that untrained clients get the best gains with three weekly training sessions (~48 hours recovery) and more well-trained clients with two weekly sessions (~72 hours recovery) for each muscle group, increasing training volume in each session (Rhea et al. 2003; Peterson et al. 2004). If the overall goal is fat loss or improvement of general fitness, resistance training must be complemented by aerobic endurance training. This has to be taken into account in order to guarantee an optimal recovery. If a HIIT session is scheduled between two resistance sessions, it is obvious that the client needs more rest days. Although much research backs up the supercompensation theory, personal trainers should use their intuition and experience in one-to-one situations. A robust approach of programme documentation is highly recommended, since it helps personal trainers determine load and recovery correctly.

Periodisation

The roots of periodisation come from Hans Selye's model, known as the *general adaptation syndrome*, which has been used by the athletic community since the late 1950s (Selye 1950). Selye identified a source of biological stress referred to as *eustress*, which denotes beneficial muscular strength and growth, as well as a distress state, which is stress that can lead to tissue damage, disease and death.

The principle of periodisation refers to the systematic process of changing one or more programme variables over time to allow the training stimulus to stay demanding and efficient (Ratamess et al. 2009). Periodisation can involve, for example, systematically alternating high loads of training with decreased loading phases to improve components of muscular fitness (e.g., maximal strength, hypertrophy and muscular endurance). Personal trainers recommend various periodisation programmes for the continuing development of their clients. Periodisation protocols are thought to optimise the continuing development of physical performance for the following reasons: Cumulative fatigue is dispersed, thereby reducing the risk for overtraining; the varying training stimuli associated with periodisation yield greater and faster gains than training at the constant intensity; and the programme remains interesting and challenging for the client, thereby improving long-term commitment.

Periodisation programmes for athletes are typically divided into three cycles of different duration: microcycle, mesocycle and macrocycle. The microcycle generally lasts up to 7 days. The mesocycle may last anywhere from 2 weeks to a few months. It can be further classified into preparation, competition, peaking and transition phases. The macrocycle refers to the overall training period, usually representing a year. It is useful to shorten this period down to 3 months, which seems to be a more realistic time frame for the client. It moreover facilitates promotion and marketing activities.

Numerous research studies have investigated physiological effects of different training volumes (total repetitions per workout) and intensities. Most research studies have demonstrated superior changes in muscle mass, strength, muscular endurance and performance of periodised over non-periodised programmes. Even over a short period of time (weeks to months), systematic variation in training volume and intensity results in greater gains compared with non-periodised programs using constant sets and repetitions (e.g., 4 sets of 10 repetitions; Fleck and Kraemer 2014; Ratamess et al. 2009).

As stated previously volume and intensity are important components of periodisation. However numerous other variables should be considered for optimal periodisation for each client: choice of exercises, order of exercises, number of muscle groups per training session, number of sets per exercise, number of exercises per muscle group, repetition range, speed of lifting and lowering the weight, rest period between sets and rest days between training the same muscle groups again.

Linear and undulating periodisation are two common systems of planned variation (see figures 15.1 and 15.2). In the linear model a training cycle begins with a high-volume, low-intensity programme, then progresses to a low-volume, high-intensity one over the coming months. Thus the linear model typically describes a progression from high-volume and low-intensity work towards decreasing volume

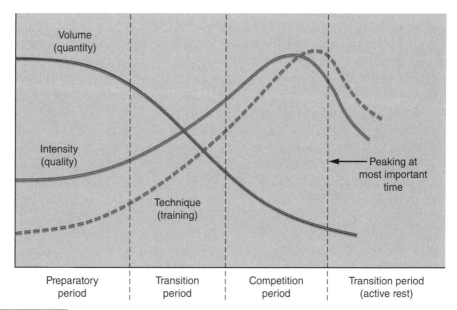

Figure 15.1 The model of linear periodisation.

Reprinted, by permission, from NSCA, 2008, Periodization, by D. Wathen et al. *Essentials of strength training and conditioning*, 3rd ed., edited by T.R. Baechle and R.W. Earle (Champaign, IL: Human Kinetics), 510.

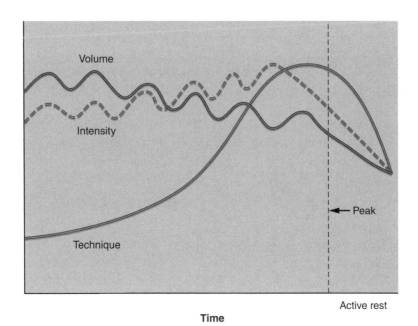

Figure 15.2 The model of undulating periodisation.

Reprinted, by permission, from NSCA, 2008, Periodization, by D. Wathen et al. *Essentials of strength training and conditioning,* 3rd ed., edited by T.R. Baechle and R.W. Earle (Champaign, IL: Human Kinetics), 510.

and increasing intensity during the different cycles. A variant of linear periodisation is the stepwise periodisation in which intensity increases and volume decreases during the training period, but volume is decreased in a stepwise fashion (e.g., repetitions are reduced from 10 to 8, 8 to 5, 5 to 2 and so on at specific time intervals; Kraemer and Fleck 2007).

In undulating periodisation training volume and intensity increase and decrease on a regular basis rather than following the linear pattern. Intensity and volume are typically shifted up and down on a weekly basis. This type of periodised loading is thought to optimise strength gains by regularly inducing training stimuli and to favour both muscle growth (high-volume training) and neural adaptations (high-intensity training).

Numerous periodisation programmes exist. Two popular and effective programmes are hypertrophy-specific training (HST) and Smolov Jr. training.

Hypertrophy-Specific Training (HST)

In HST, a full-body programme is performed three times weekly with 7 to 10 exercises and one or two sets of each exercise (see the example in table 15.2). The programme contains three linearly periodised 2-week microcycles with increasing intensity across the cycles. The

Table 15.2   Example of Hypertrophy-Specific Training (HST)

Weeks 1+2					
Day 1	Day 2	Day 3	Day 4	Day 5	Day 6
75% of 15RM	80% of 15RM	85% of 15RM	90% of 15RM	95% of 15RM	100% of 15RM
Weeks 3+4					
Day 1	Day 2	Day 3	Day 4	Day 5	Day 6
75% of 10RM	80% of 10RM	85% of 10RM	90% of 10RM	95% of 10RM	100% of 10RM
Weeks 5+6					
Day 1	Day 2	Day 3	Day 4	Day 5	Day 6
75% of 5RM	80% of 5RM	85% of 5RM	90% of 5RM	95% of 5RM	100% of 5RM

programme requires that 15RM, 10RM and 5RM in each exercise are known.

Smolov Jr.

This programme effectively increases maximal strength and combines the principles of undulation, progression and concentrated loading. The programme contains four weekly training sessions, using both high volume and high intensity (see the example in table 15.3). The intensities are based on knowledge of current 1RM. The programme is primarily suited for one or two compound exercises where proper form can be maintained even in a fatigued state (e.g., bench press, pull-down, leg press), whereas rows, curls and dead lifts are less well suited due to increased risk of injury.

If 1RM is more than 150 kilograms, 10 kilograms are added in the second week and 15 kilograms in the third week. If a client follows a Smolov Jr. cycle for the bench press, they should not do any additional pressing and isolation work for pressing muscles during the 4 weeks.

Table 15.3   Example of a Smolov Jr. Microcycle

	Day 1	Day 2	Day 3	Day 4
Week 1	6 × 6 @ 70%*	7 × 5 @ 75%	8 × 4 @ 80%	10 × 3 @ 85%
Week 2	6 × 6 @ 70% + 5 kg	7 × 5 @ 75% + 5 kg	8 × 4 @ 80% + 5 kg	10 × 3 @ 85% + 5 kg
Week 3	6 × 6 @ 70% + 7.5 kg	7 × 5 @ 75% + 7.5 kg	8 × 4 @ 80% + 7.5 kg	10 × 3 @ 85% + 7.5 kg
Week 4	OFF			

*The workout is read as the number of sets of the number of repetitions at the percent of the 1RM for the exercise.

Examples of Exercise Programming

The following case studies describe a 3-month macrocycle for clients with a variety of fitness statuses (Klein 1997). The examples provided illuminate conditions, limitations and programming that are commonly presented to personal trainers who work with the general public.

Case 1: Beginner, Slightly Overweight

The client's goal is to improve overall fitness and lose body weight. Within the recommended time frame the personal trainer should divide the 3-month macrocycle into three 4-week periods. The first weeks should include familiarisation with equipment and machines and teaching elemental movements (light weights, 15 to 20 repetitions, approximately 30 percent of the theoretical maximum weight) and low-intensity aerobic endurance training (15 to 30 minutes) for fat burning or as a basic training.

The following 4-week period continues with resistance training, applying light intensity with 12 to 15 repetitions and 40 to 50 percent of the maximum weight. Technique improvement comes first. In addition, personal trainers should include 20 to 30 minutes of aerobic endurance training with moderate intensity using either the duration or interval method. The last time period encompasses light hypertrophy training (10 to 12 repetitions, 50 to 60 percent of the maximum weight) and longer aerobic endurance training of 30 to 45 minutes using the Fartlek method (see chapter 7).

Case 2: Returnee

This macrocycle is divided into a 6-week starting period, followed by 2-week and 4-week periods. The 6 weeks include resistance training as basic training with 12 to 15 repetitions and 60 to 70 percent of the maximum weight and aerobic endurance training with moderate intensity (20 to 30 minutes). Use of the interval method is possible. Next personal trainers should use 2 weeks of intramuscular co-ordination training (3 to 6 repetitions with 80 to 90 percent of the maximum weight), followed by a short aerobic endurance training (10 to 15 minutes) aiming for active recovery. The last period (4 weeks) contains light hypertrophy training (10 to 12 repetitions, 40 to 50 percent of the maximum weight), complemented by moderate aerobic endurance training (20 to 30 minutes). If body fat is an issue, it is helpful to move to duration of 30 to 45 minutes with low intensity.

Case 3: Very Obese Client

If personal trainers work with very obese clients, the first and foremost aspect in the programming is respect. Personal trainers must always appreciate the client's decision to overcome their current situation, because in their daily life these people are very often confronted with mockery. In this regard the personal trainer has to use their psychological competencies more than the other, more obvious skills related to exercising, programming and so forth. In terms of exercise programming the alliance between massive overweight and poor fitness levels significantly affects the first weeks or even months. Any kind of body-weight exercise will be problematic except squat variants with a partial range of motion. Personal trainers in this case need to involve exercises that allow easy adaptations with regard to the limited physical capacity of the client. Exercises like leg press, lat pull-down and bench press variants fulfil this requirement and, in addition, activate different muscles and joints simultaneously, which then leads to a better overall conditioning effect. Moreover co-ordination, one of the main sport motor functions, is trained as well. The selection of aerobic endurance training modes is also limited. Due to the client's body weight and its impact on the joints and bones, jogging is not an adequate option. Walking on the treadmill or outside and using the recumbent machine or stationary bike are the most obvious alternatives. Personal trainers can apply a low-intensity interval method for all three of these alternatives in order to aim for an acceptable workout duration. Particularly for this target group, awareness and sensitivity are key, since very obese clients tend to quit the programme if they experience any kind of discomfort or overload. Thus success primarily lies in the personal trainer's motivational skills and talent to correctly interpret the signals clients send.

Conclusion

In order to achieve a desired outcome from a training programme, personal trainers must manage training intensity, training volume and exercise order. For the well-trained client, personal trainers can apply a number of advanced techniques to increase the training stimuli. Further it is beneficial to periodise the programming so that intensity, training volume and recovery are systematically varied over time. This includes resistance as well as aerobic endurance training. Although planning and programming must be grounded on current research, personal trainers need intuition and an instinctive feeling for each client to deliver the optimal programme. A gapless documentation of every detail in the programme such as weights, intensity and the client's mood is mandatory. Moreover it is crucial to decide which sessions should be supervised and unsupervised. This depends on the complexity of each session. Resistance training should be prioritised in this regard, especially if it aims for compound movements, which require a permanent observation by the personal trainer. Low-intensity, steady-state aerobic endurance sessions are on the other end of the scale. Clients are able to check their own heart rate and maintain a certain range for a defined period of time. Personal training is a very individualised experience. Hence planning and programming looks different from client to client. Personal trainers should not make the mistake of underestimating the relevance of psychological aspects when it comes to planning and delivering the ideal programme. Listening to the client is always the first choice.

Appendix

European Qualifications Framework (EQF) Level 4: Personal Trainer

Introductory Information

What does level 4 mean at EQF?

Level of the EQF	Knowledge is described as theoretical and/or factual.	Skills are described as cognitive (involving the use of logical, intuitive and creative thinking) and practical (involving manual dexterity and the use of methods, materials, tools and instruments).	Competence is described in terms of responsibility and autonomy.
The learning outcomes relevant to Level 4 are	Factual and theoretical knowledge in broad contexts within a field of work or study	A range of cognitive and practical skills required to generate solutions to specific problems in a field of work or study	Exercise self-management within the guidelines of work or study contexts that are usually predictable, but are subject to change. Supervise the routine work of others, taking some responsibility for the evaluation and improvement of work or study activities.

What does level 4 mean at Fitness QF?

EQF Level	Occupation	EHFA Standards	Target Audience
Level 4	Personal Trainer[1]	EHFA Level 4	General Population

It is assumed that the Personal Trainer (Level 4 EQF) will have acquired all knowledge required to work as a Fitness Assistant and Instructor as identified in the EuropeActive Fitness Assistant Guide (Level 2 EQF, Fitness Assistant) and Instructor Guide (Level 3 EQF, Instructor). Thus, these standards should be read in conjunction with *EuropeActive's Foundations for Exercise Professionals* and *EuropeActive's Foundations for Fitness Instructors*, both published by Human Kinetics.

EQF Level 4

Occupational Title

Personal Trainer

Job Purpose

Coach clients individually according to their fitness needs, through an agreed exercise/ physical activity plan and assist with behavioural change.

Occupational Description

A personal trainer's role includes designing, implementing and evaluating exercise/physical activity programmes for a range of individual clients by collecting and analysing client information to ensure the effectiveness of personal exercise programmes. A personal trainer should also actively encourage potential clients/members to participate in and adhere to regular exercise/physical activity programmes, employing appropriate motivational strategies to achieve this.

Occupational Roles

The personal trainer should be able to:

1. Collect information relating to individual clients
2. Carry out fitness assessments to establish client fitness and skill level
3. Analyse information relating to individual clients
4. Identify, agree and review short-, medium- and long-term goals to ensure the effectiveness of exercise programmes
5. Provide a range of exercise programmes in accordance with the needs of the clients by applying principles of exercise programming
6. Make best use of the environment in which clients are exercising
7. Provide clients with accurate information on the principles of nutrition and weight management

8. Develop and apply strategies to motivate clients to join and adhere to an exercise programme

9. Deliver good customer service and be a positive role model at all times and keep up to date with industry developments

10. Promote healthy activities and related strategies for daily living to clients/members

11. Make the appropriate decisions relating to clients and their programmes/goals and, where required, refer the client to a more appropriate professional

12. Work within the parameters given at Level 3, recognizing the standards and professional limitations that this provides, refer-ring to appropriate members of staff for guidance and support.

EuropeActive Level 4 Personal Trainer: Knowledge Areas

Role of the Personal Trainer	Functional Anatomy	Physiology	Nutrition
Psychosocial Aspects of Health and Fitness	Health and Fitness Assessment: Collecting and Analysing Information	Training Adaptation and Exercise Planning and Programming	

Section 1: Role of the Personal Trainer

Section Overview

- Knowledge and understanding of the basic roles of the exercise professional as a personal trainer
- Knowledge and understanding of the principles that underpin personal training and how personal training differs from other types of physical activity/exercise instruction

Content Summary and Learning Outcomes:

1.1 Professionalism, Code of Practice/Ethics/National Standards and Guidelines

Learners should demonstrate knowledge and understanding of:

- The ethical requirements that are intrinsic to the Personal Trainer role as stated in the EuropeActive and EREPS code of ethical practice (for more visit www.ereps.eu)

1.2 Presentation

Learners should demonstrate knowledge and understanding of:

- Basic procedures to introduce him/herself to new clients
- General rules for customer care
- The basic principles of customer care to include perceived benefits
- The methods and practices that contribute to effective customer care
- The skills of effective customer care: *communication, body language, negotiation*

1.3 Communication

Learners should demonstrate knowledge and understanding of:

- The personal communication skills necessary to develop rapport in order to motivate individuals to begin exercise, adhere to exercise and return to exercise early
- Building rapport:
  □ The importance of connecting people: body language: posture, eye contact, facial expression, vocal tonality (tempo, intensity, voice inflection)
  □ Primacy effects: smiling, mimicking. . . .
  □ Using sensory communication (visual, auditory, kinesthetic pattern) to improve communication and orientation of the client
  □ The use of open-ended questioning, reflecting answering
- Motivational interviewing:
  □ Developing 'importance', 'confidence' and 'readiness'
  □ Dealing with resistance to change
  □ Using open-ended question, reflecting answering, summarizing
  □ Technique of decisional balance sheet
  □ Removing barriers, problem solving and enhancing benefits of practicing physical activity
- Motivational strategies:
  □ The most important and effective behavioural strategies to enhance exercise and health behaviour change (e.g., reinforcement, goal setting, social support, problem solving, reinforcement strategies, self-monitoring, etc.)
  □ Knowing about the different stages of change of the trans-theoretical model Prochaska and DiClemente, being able to use basic strategies for different stages

- Using the sensory representational system (visual, auditory, kinesthetic) to optimize an individual's training session
- Definition and practical examples of extrinsic and intrinsic reinforcement
- Relapse prevention: planning, problem solving, identifying and changing negative thinking

1.4 Health Promotion

Learners should demonstrate knowledge and understanding of:

- The cardiovascular, muscular and flexibility related benefits of physical activity and the significance of these benefits in reducing risk of disease
- Appropriate exercise activity required for health benefits and fitness benefits
- The barriers and motivators to exercise participation
- The exercise guidelines for health, well being and physical fitness
- The exercise continuum for different levels of physical activity to include relative benefits
- The agencies involved in promoting activity for health in your country
- How to promote a healthy lifestyle: Nutrition, other opportunities for physical activity in everyday life, smoking

1.5 Plan and Deliver Personal Training

Learners should demonstrate knowledge and understanding of:

- The principles that underpin personal training and how personal training differs from other types of physical activity instruction
- The difference between planning supervised and unsupervised activities and how to build these into a timetable of sessions
- The types of environment within which personal training may be delivered and how to make best use of these
- Specific health and safety issues about delivering personal training in an environment not designed for physical activity instruction
- How to improvise effective activities with the client according to the resources available
- The importance of maintaining frequent contact with the client, including between sessions

- The proactive role of the personal trainer regarding the adaptation process in each individual especially at the beginning of the training programme
- The importance of providing a proper dose response relationship according to the level of the individual
- The importance of regular and planned communication strategy regarding the training adaptation process

Section 2: Functional Anatomy

2.1 Functional Kinesiology/Biomechanics

Learners should demonstrate knowledge and understanding of:

- The body's three anatomical axes and planes including the terms frontal (coronal), sagittal and transverse
- The classification of joints in the human body (fibrous, cartilaginous and synovial) focusing on their functional significance including examples of each type and sub-types of joint
- The importance of ensuring that movement at all joints is kept in the correct planes throughout exercise performance for prevention of ligament strain and potential risk of injury (e.g., at shoulder joint, inappropriate biomechanics can place a strain on the rotator cuff muscles increasing risk of osteo-ligamentus injury)
- Stability and movement within each type of joint
- Classification of bones—to include long, short, flat, irregular, sesamoid, relating structure to function
- Role of osteoblasts and osteoclasts, hormonal contribution in bone density
- Bone density and its relation to resistance training activities
- Long- and short-term effects of exercise on bone to include osteoporosis
- Articulations and the joint movements possible. To include the following movement terms with examples: flexion, extension, hyperextension, adduction, abduction, elevation, depression, protraction, retraction, lateral flexion, horizontal flexion and extension, plantar flexion, dorsiflexion, internal and external rotation, circumduction, pronation, supination, eversion and inversion
- The main bones and their implications for vital functions and movements
- The vertebral column: structure and function—role of curves

- The importance of maintaining the correct degree of spinal curvature at the cervical, lumbar and thoracic vertebra regarding weight-bearing and biomechanical efficiency and for the transmission of stress, caused by impact, through the pelvic girdle, kinetic chain and muscle synergies
- Abnormal degrees of curvature in the spine (lordosis, kyphosis and scoliosis) and their importance to exercise safety and the design of appropriate activities
- The high risk of shoulder joint displacement and increased scapular stabilising role of the surrounding synergistic musculature and ligaments
- The potential for sprains and ligamentus damage increased by excessive non-functional movement during activities, such as running
- The main structural and physiological characteristics and functions of the osseous connective tissues to include the periosteum, ligaments (dense regular collagenous/elastic fibres), joint capsule (dense irregular, elastic, collagenous), fasciae
- The structure of ligaments and their tensile strength related to fibre direction and their sensitivity to shearing forces and tearing
- Biomechanical principles of movement—to include $1^{st,}$ 2nd and 3rd class levers with examples (e.g., calf raises for 2nd class lever and flexion of the elbow for 3rd class lever)
- Biomechanical implications of different centres of gravity in relation to posture and patterns of adiposity
- Open and closed chain kinetic movements with examples of each and a consideration of their advantages and disadvantages

2.2 Muscles

Learners should demonstrate knowledge and understanding of:

- The three types of muscle in the human body (skeletal, smooth, cardiac)
- The gross anatomy and structure of a skeletal muscle and its connective tissue
- The connective tissue of muscle merging into tendons composed of regular collagenous filaments
- Muscle shape and fibre arrangement including directional forces and line of pull (uni-pennate, bi-pennate, multi-pennate)
- The role of proprioceptors of tendons

- The interaction between the contractile filaments of muscle (actine and myosine)
- The role of a motor unit (e.g., the nerve and the muscle fibres which it innervates) in providing an 'action potential' to create fine or course muscle control
- The structural features and characteristics of Type 1 (slow twitch) and Type 2A (fast twitch/intermediate) and Type 2B fibres and the implications of exercise intensity on the recruitment sequence of different motor unit types
- The different types of muscular contractions (concentric, eccentric, isometric, isotonic and isokinetic)
- The effect of each type of muscular contraction on training adaptations and the way muscles can be influenced by different training modalities (e.g., body position in relation to gravity, aqua workouts and partner work)
- The likely relationship between delayed onset of muscular soreness (D.O.M.S.) and both eccentric, concentric and isometric muscle work
- The major muscles of the body defining their starting points in terms of the bones they originate from (though in most cases NOT the exact anatomical part of the bone), the joints that they cross and the bones that they insert onto (finishing point)
- The joint actions as a result of muscular action
- A range of actions and activities, the agonists, antagonists, main synergists and fixators
- The functional role of abdominal muscles in synergy with other muscles on the trunk, rib cage, pelvis and vertebral column
- Role of muscles like gluteus and latissimus dorsi and thoraco-lumbar fasciae
- The importance of correct involvement of the hip flexor muscle, iliopsoas, in core stability training
- Role played by hip flexor muscles iliopsoas complex and pelvic floor in core training
- Short- and long-term effects of exercise on muscles

Section 3: Physiology

3.1 Energy Systems

Learners should demonstrate knowledge and understanding of:

- The three energy systems used for the production of ATP in working muscle—the alactic anaerobic phosphocreatine (PC) system, the anaerobic lactate system and the aerobic system

- The effect of the type of exercise, intensity, duration, fitness levels, nutritional level on the three energy systems
- The way to use the three energy systems in correlation to the goal of the client
- The way to use acute variables during training to create the different energy systems
- The terms aerobic and anaerobic threshold
- Effects of interval training and EPOC effects on the metabolism
- The ability of the body to burn fat throughout a range of intensities (not just low intensity) e.g., if the aerobic threshold is raised you can utilize fat more effectively at higher intensities
- The relationship between METs and kilocalories and the prediction of calorie expenditure based on body weight, exercise MET level and duration with examples of different activities and their MET values
- The methods of monitoring exercise intensity—to include; RPE - 6 to 20 or 0 to 10 - talk test, heart rate monitoring (age related and Karvonen), the benefits and limitations of each method
- The use and amounts of energy nutrients at different intensities

3.2 Cardiorespiratory System

Learners should demonstrate knowledge and understanding of:

- The anatomy of the heart to include the names and location of the heart valves, muscular component and flow of blood through the heart
- The cardiac cycle and the terms stroke volume (amount of blood pumped per beat) and cardiac output (amount of blood pumped per minute = stroke volume × beats per minute)
- The structure, function and characteristics of arteries, arterioles, veins, venules and capillaries
- The effect of physical activity on cardiovascular system
- Understanding the effect of medication for the cardiovascular system and their impact on training
- The respiratory system: description and function
- The relationship between the cardiovascular system and respiratory system and how regular physical activity impacts them
- The passage of inhaled air from the atmosphere to cellular level and back
- Healthy lifestyle choices and their positive effect on cardiorespiratory tissues, e.g., the effects of smoking or alcohol consumption

- Short- and long-term effects of exercise on the cardiorespiratory system to include short term – increase in heart rate, increase in breathing rate, effects of building up of CO_2 in bloodstream. Long term effects including increase in stroke volume, lower resting heart rate, reduced risk of heart disease, reduction of high blood pressure, improved blood cholesterol, reduction of body fat and increased everyday function etc.
- Coronary heart disease and risk factors that can manipulate it such as smoking, high blood pressure, high blood cholesterol, physical inactivity, diabetes mellitus, family history, age, stress, obesity

3.3 Nervous and Endocrine System

Learners should demonstrate knowledge and understanding of:

- The main responsibilities of the nervous system to include:
  - Sensory Input—monitoring events in and outside the body
  - Interpretation—analysing data
  - Motor Output—response to incoming data
- The two parts of the nervous system– the central nervous system (CNS) incorporating the brain and spinal cord and the peripheral nervous system (PNS) consisting of all nerves extending from the spinal cord, to include:
- The role of the CNS in receiving input from the sense organs and receptors about the state of both the external and internal environment, collating all of the information and sending out messages via the motor neurons of the PNS to effectors (muscles and glands)
- The PNS and its divisions into somatic and autonomic branches
- The somatic branch terminating at the neuromuscular junction controlling movement under voluntary control
- The role of the autonomic nervous system in controlling cardiac and smooth muscle, the endocrine glands that secrete hormones and other organs, thereby regulating their activity
- The two opposing branches (to include the neurotransmitters and receptors) and their roles, e.g., sympathetic nerves speed up responses (e.g. heart rate) and mobilise energy stores to get us ready for action, parasympathetic nerves slow things down and are more active during periods of calm and relaxation
- Regular activity for the nervous system, which enhances hardwire neuromuscular connections and improves all of the features of motor fitness such as reaction times, balance, spatial awareness and coordination, etc.

- Description of hormonal response to exercise and their catabolic and anabolic role
- Link between type of exercise intensity and hormonal reaction for specific goals like in a weight loss, muscle building or wellness programme
- Role of cortisol and side effects of too high production

Section 4: Nutrition

Learners should demonstrate knowledge and understanding of:

- The dietary role and common dietary sources for each of the six main nutrients (carbohydrate, fat, protein, vitamins, minerals, water)
- Balance between saturated and unsaturated fatty acid and effects on health
- The importance of right intake of essential fatty acids (Omega3 and 6) and their effects on health
- The role of vitamins and minerals in cells' metabolic process
- The role and desirable levels of total cholesterol, HDLs and LDLs in the body, including the total cholesterol/HDL ratio
- Examples of food items in each of the four basic food groups
- Examples of food items for vitamins and minerals intake
- The components of the energy balance (basal metabolic rate, thermic effect of food, physical activity level)
- Methods to estimate calories requirements
- How to develop a healthy, balanced way of eating
- Healthy eating patterns
- How dietary intake influences health; how lack of micronutrients (vitamins and minerals) influences health
- Lifestyle advice, to include use of tobacco, alcohol, caffeine (current government guidelines)
- How some medical conditions (e.g., CHD, diabetes mellitus, obesity, osteoporosis) may be impacted by nutrition (general advice)
- Energy needs for different activities/sports/fitness plans
- The role of carbohydrate, fat and protein as fuels for aerobic and anaerobic exercise
- Safe and effective advices about eating pattern for weight (fat) loss/gain; energy balance; appropriate 'weight'-loss goals
- Appropriate referral/advice organisations
- Analysis of current weight-loss fads and popular diets

Section 5: Psychosocial Aspects of Health and Fitness

Learners should demonstrate knowledge and understanding of:

- The different underlying motives for goal setting (internal & external motivation)
- The psychological aspects of health and fitness, which are influential to health and fitness behaviour change (e.g., behaviour modification, reinforcement, goal setting, social support and peer pressure, etc.)
- The application of basic cognitive-behavioural intervention such as shaping, goal setting, motivation, cueing, problem solving, reinforcement strategies and self-monitoring
- Motives and barriers, perceived and actual, to participation in physical activity (e.g., relapse prevention model, self liberation, social liberation, etc.)
- Appropriate models for change such as the 'Prochaska & DiClemente' models and the characteristics of an individual at each stage and the appropriate interventions/strategies at each stage. (e.g., decisional balance, self efficacy, fitness testing, stimulus control, reinforcement management and counter conditioning, etc.)
- The selection of an appropriate behavioural goal and the suggested method to evaluate goal achievement for each stage of change
- Signs and symptoms of stress, the effects of stress on health and strategies for dealing with stress

Section 6: Health and Fitness Assessment: Collecting and Analysing Information

6.1 Components of Fitness

Learners should demonstrate knowledge and understanding of:

- The three different somatotypes (endomorphic, ectomorphic and mesomorphic) focusing on the implications of each body type for exercise capacity and ability to alter body shape
- Anatomical and hormonal differences concerning males and females and their influence on safe, effective and appropriate physical activity
- The health and skill related components of total fitness and their definitions to include:

□ Health-related:
  - Muscular strength
  - Muscular endurance
  - Cardiorespiratory endurance (heart and lungs)
  - Flexibility
  - Body composition
□ Skill-related:
  - Balance (static and dynamic)
  - Coordination
  - Reaction time
  - Power
  - Agility

6.2 Collecting and Analysing Information

Learners should demonstrate knowledge and understanding of:

- Appropriate information relevant to the ability to negotiate goals that are specific, measurable, achievable, realistic, time bound to plan and carry out safe and effective programmes to enable thorough evaluation of planning options

- Correct screening procedures for:
  □ Physical; previous and current level of activity and interests. Evaluation of current levels of all components of fitness—muscular strength, muscular endurance, cardio-pulmonary fitness, flexibility and motor skills (balance & coordination)
  □ Psychological; motivation to participate, perceived and actual barriers to participation, stage of readiness to participate and stated future goals and aspirations
  □ Medical; health history, current health status, particularly in relation to risk factors for heart disease, the identification of medical conditions that would necessitate medical clearance and past and present injuries and disabilities
  □ Lifestyle; work patterns, eating patterns, relevant personal circumstances, likes, dislikes and preferences toward physical activity

- The screening process to identify: risk factors for coronary heart disease; factors that limit the ability to participate/achieve goals; those requiring a referral to an appropriate medical professional or other clinician or medically supervised exercise programme

- How to adapt basic programmes for participants with particular needs including: sedentary, recovering from injury, over-trained, peak performer, sport-specific performer, obese

- Appropriate use of:
  - ☐ Medical questionnaires: Physical Activity Readiness Questionnaire (PAR-Q), medical clearance, informed consent, psychological questionnaires, lifestyle questionnaires, etc.
  - ☐ Other professionals: GP's, physiotherapists, neuromuscular therapists, consultants, etc.
  - ☐ Fitness assessments: cardiorespiratory fitness, muscular strength, muscular endurance, flexibility, postural analysis, body composition, contraindications and limitation for testing
  - ☐ Postural assessment—to include:
    - Optimal postural alignment
    - Postural deficiencies and postural deviations
    - Factors affecting posture
    - Posture and client health
    - Static and dynamic postural analysis
    - Selection of suitable assessments
    - Factors to assess
    - Limitations of personal trainer
    - Appropriate health and fitness assessments specific to the client needs

Section 7: Training Adaptation and Exercise Planning and Programming

7.1 Training Adaptation

Learners should demonstrate knowledge and understanding of:

- The principles of adaptation and modification for each component:
- The continuum between muscular strength (predominantly type 2 fibres) and muscular endurance (type 1 fibres) and neuromuscular efficiency
- Muscular strength influenced by use of high resistance and low repetitions so that motor unit recruitment is maximised and contractile limits are reached
- Muscular endurance enhanced by lower resistance loads and higher repetitions resulting in the buildup of lactic acid and inducing inhibition of further muscle contraction
- Increased endurance capacity in muscles developed between exercise sessions by the acquisition of increased numbers of mitochondria, oxidative enzymes and capillaries leading to increased oxidative ability within muscles

- The repetition ranges for strength, power, endurance and muscle hypertrophy
- The range of heart rate training zone models (e.g., aerobic training zone, fitness zone) for developing aerobic and anaerobic capacity
- Interval, Fartlek principles and practical application
- The principles of training including specificity, progressive overload, reversibility, adaptability, individuality and recovery time
- The effects of health-related physical activities, to include resistance training (e.g., improved posture, reduced risk of joint and soft tissue injuries, increased bone density, improved neuromuscular efficiency, etc.), cardiorespiratory training (reduced risk of CHD, improved body composition, etc.) and range of motion training
- The principles of periodized training programmes in developing components of fitness
- The use of short-, medium- and long-term goals (micro, meso and macro-cycles)
- The use of volume vs. intensity through the periodization stages
- The various methods of range of motion (flexibility) training, the advantages and disadvantages of each, including static, ballistic, dynamic and proprioceptive neuromuscular techniques (including myotactic) to facilitate increased range of motion
- The role of the muscle spindle cells and the golgi tendon organs in these mechanisms (including myotactic reflexes, contract relax, antagonist, contract)
- The current ACSM or other recognized international guidelines for developing the different components of fitness, emphasizing the distinction between activity for health and exercise from evidence-based information
- The importance of adequate rest phases between training loads and the signs and symptoms of overtraining
- The principles frequency, intensity, time, type for health- and skill-related components of fitness

7.2 Exercise Planning and Programming

Learners should demonstrate knowledge and understanding of:

- The principles of overload, specificity, progression and general adaptations and how they relate to exercise programming and a variety of individual wants, goals and needs

- The signs and symptoms of excessive effort that would indicate a change of intensity
- The ability to recognize correct exercise technique to include appropriate positioning, correct settings for CV machines and general safety considerations
- The ability to modify exercises appropriate to a variety of individual needs
- Training variables to include:
  □ Choice of exercises
  □ Sequence of exercise
  □ Resistance and repetitions
  □ Number of sets
  □ Rest between sets (recovery)
  □ Speed of movement
  □ Type of muscle contraction
  □ Duration of session
  □ Rest between sessions
  □ Volume of training
  □ Split routines
- The use of the above variables to develop strength, endurance, hypertrophy, speed, power
- The advantages and disadvantages of exercising at various intensities for: sedentary (untrained), experienced (trained), high performers (well trained)
- Calculations of repetition maximums (1RM – 10RM)
- Commonly used resistance training systems evidence-based to include:
  □ Single set training
  □ Circuit resistance training
  □ Basic sets
  □ Super setting (agonist/antagonist)
  □ Super setting two exercises for same muscle
  □ Pyramid systems
  □ Forced repetitions
- Commonly used cardiorespiratory training systems to include:
  □ Interval
  □ Fartlek
  □ Aerobic
  □ Anaerobic
  □ Peripheral heart flow training
- The suitability of each training system for the client, when fitness levels and goals are considered

- Safe and effective use of equipment
- The basic principles of progressive programming
- The reasons for using periodization
- The basic principles of periodization to include: the main two variables, volume and intensity
- Macrocycles (long term), mesocycle (medium term), microcycles (short term)
- Teaching strategies to enhance the individual performance
- Appropriate methods to adjust programmes to meet the changing needs and circumstances of clients
- Methods of monitoring exercise intensity to include:
  - Maximum heart rate formula
  - Rate of Perceived Exertion (RPE) scales, both 6–20 and 1–10
  - Metabolic equivalents (METs)
  - Kilocalories per hour (Kcal/hr)
  - Visual assessment and verbal assessment (talk test)
- Understand their own limitations and when to refer clients to other relevant professionals, e.g., exercise specialist, medical professional

The full version of EuropeActive's EQF-level 4 Standards Personal Trainer can be downloaded at www.ehfa standards.eu/?q=node/12.

References

Preface

U.S. Bureau of Labor Statistics. 2010. Available from: www.bls.gov.

Chapter 1

American College of Sports Medicine (ACSM). 2007. *ACSM's Resources for the Personal Trainer.* 2nd ed. Baltimore: Lippincott Williams & Wilkins.

Earle, R.W., and T.R. Baechle. 2003. *NSCA's Essentials of Personal Training.* Champaign, IL: Human Kinetics.

Horn, D. 2011. *Personal Training in Deutschland; Daten, Fakten, Zahlen.* Karlsruhe, Germany: Health and Beauty Business Media.

Kronsteiner, M. 2010. "Motivation für Personaltraining im Fitnessstudio." Master's thesis, University of Vienna. Available from: http://othes.univie.ac.at/10688/1/2010-06-28_0152147.pdf

Lucassen J., M. Van Bottenburg, and J. Van Hoecke. 2006. *Sneller, Hoger, Sterker, Beter: Kwaliteitsmanagement in de Sport.* 2nd ed. Nieuwegein, Netherlands: Arko Sportsmedia.

Melton, D.I., J.A. Katula, and K.M. Mustian. 2008. The current state of personal training: An industry perspective of personal trainers in a small Southeast community. *Journal of Strength and Conditioning Research* 22(3): 883–889.

Melton, D.I., T.K. Dail, J.A. Katula, and K.M. Mustian. 2010. The current state of personal training: Managers' perspectives. *Journal of Strength and Conditioning Research* 24(11): 3173–3179.

Middelkamp, J., and G. Willemsen, eds. 2010. *Personal training in Europa.* Waalwijk, Netherlands: LAPT.

Rieger, T., F. Naclerio, A. Jimènez, and J. Moody, eds. 2015. *EuropeActive's Foundations for Exercise Professionals.* Champaign, IL: Human Kinetics.

Chapter 2

Donnelly, J.E., S.N. Blair, J.M. Jakicic, M.M. Manore, J.W. Rankin, and B.K. Smith. 2009. American College of Sports Medicine position stand. Appropriate physical activity intervention strategies for weight loss and prevention of weight regain for adults. *Medicine and Science in Sports and Exercise* 41(2): 459–471.

Garber, C.E., B. Blissmer, M.R. Deschenes, B.A. Franklin, M.J. Lamonte, I.M. Lee et al. 2011. American College of Sports Medicine position stand. Quantity and quality of exercise for developing and maintaining cardiorespiratory, musculoskeletal, and neuromotor fitness in apparently healthy adults: Guidance for prescribing exercise. *Medicine and Science in Sports and Exercise* 43(7): 1334–1359.

Hines, E. 2008. *Fitness Swimming.* 2nd ed. Champaign, IL: Human Kinetics.

Kieß, E. 2012. *Personal Training. Idee, Konzept, Marketing.* Saarbrücken, Germany: Akademiker Verlag.

Klein, V. 1997. *Privat-Trainer.* Arnsberg, Germany: Novagenics.

Kraemer, W.J., and N.A. Ratamess. 2004. Fundamentals of resistance training: Progression and exercise prescription. *Medicine and Science in Sports and Exercise* 36(4): 674–688.

Kraemer, W.J., K. Adams, E. Cafarelli, G.A. Dudley, C. Dooly, M.S. Feigenbaum et al. 2009. American College of Sports Medicine position stand. Progression models in resistance training for healthy adults. *Medicine and Science in Sports and Exercise* 41(3): 687–708.

Kuhr, E.M., R.A. Ribeiro, L.E. Rohde, and C.A. Polanczyk. 2011. Cost-effectiveness of supervised exercise therapy in heart failure patients. *Value Health* 14(5): 100–107.

Mazzetti, S.A., W.J. Kraemer, J.S. Volek, N.D. Duncan, N.A. Ratamess, A.L. Gomez et al. 2000. The influence of direct supervision of resistance training on strength performance. *Medicine and Science in Sports and Exercise* 32(6): 1175–1184.

Middelkamp, J., and T. Rieger. 2013. *EHFA's Retention Report 2013. A Comprehensive Understanding of Member Retention in Fitness Clubs.* Nijmegen, Netherlands: Black Box.

Olney, S.J., J. Nymark, B. Brouwer, E. Culham, A. Day, J. Heard et al. 2006. A randomized controlled trial of supervised versus unsupervised exercise programs for ambulatory stroke survivors. *Stroke* 37(2): 476–481.

Ratamess, N.A., A.D. Faigenbaum, J.R. Hoffman, and J. Kang. 2008. Self-selected resistance training intensity in healthy women: The influence of a personal trainer. *Journal of Strength and Conditioning Research* 22(1): 103–111.

Rieger, T. 2015a. Building rapport and customer care. In *EuropeActive's Foundations for Exercise Professionals*, edited by T. Rieger, F. Naclerio, A. Jimènez, and J. Moody. Champaign, IL: Human Kinetics.

Rieger, T. 2015b. Customer service. In *EuropeActive's Essentials for Fitness Instructors*, edited by R. Santos-Rocha, T. Rieger, and A. Jimènez. Champaign, IL: Human Kinetics.

Saetre, T., E. Enoksen, T. Lyberg, E. Stranden, J.J. Jorgensen, J.O. Sundhagen et al. 2011. Supervised exercise training reduces plasma levels of the endothelial inflammatory markers E-selectin and ICAM-I in patients with peripheral arterial disease. *Angiology* 62(4): 301–305.

Sovndal, S. 2013. *Fitness Cycling.* Champaign, IL: Human Kinetics.

Van Asselt, A.D., S.P. Nicolai, M.A. Joore, M.H. Prins, and J.A. Teijink. 2011. Cost-effectiveness of exercise therapy in patients with intermittent claudication: Supervised exercise therapy versus a 'go home and walk' advice. *European Journal of Vascular and Endovascular Surgery* 41(1): 97–103.

Chapter 3

American College of Sports Medicine (ACSM). 2013. *ACSM's Guidelines for Exercise Testing and Prescription.* 9th ed. Baltimore: Lippincott Williams & Wilkins.

Ashford, S., J. Edmunds, and D.P. French. 2010. What is the best way to change self-efficacy to promote lifestyle and recreational physical activity? A systematic review with meta-analysis. *British Journal of Health Psychology* 15(Pt 2): 265–288. doi:10.1348/135910709X461752.

Bandura, A. 1977. Self-efficacy: Toward a unifying theory of behavioral change. *Psychological Review* 84(2): 191–215.

Barr-Anderson, D.J., M. AuYoung, M.C. Whitt-Glover, B.A. Glenn, and A.K. Yancey. 2011. Integration of short bouts of physical activity into organizational routine: A systematic review of the literature. *American Journal of Preventive Medicine* 40(1): 76–93. doi:10.1016/j.amepre.2010.09.033.

Bonelli, S. 2000. *Step Training. ACE's Group Fitness Specialty Series.* San Diego: American Council on Exercise.

Brooks, D. 2004. *The Complete Book of Personal Training*. Champaign, IL: Human Kinetics.

Canadian Society of Exercise Physiology (CSEP). 2010. *The Canadian Physical Activity, Fitness and Lifestyle Approach*. Vancouver, BC: Author.

Cancelliere, C., J.D. Cassidy, C. Ammendolia, and P. Cote. 2011. Are workplace health promotion programs effective at improving presenteeism in workers? A systematic review and best evidence synthesis of the literature. *BMC Public Health* 11: 395. doi:10.1186/1471-2458-11-395.

Clark, A.M., L. Hartling, B. Vandermeer, and F.A. McAlister. 2005. Meta-analysis: Secondary prevention programs for patients with coronary artery disease. *Annals of Internal Medicine* 143(9): 659–672.

Cloostermans, L., M.B. Bekkers, E. Uiters, and K.I. Proper. 2014. The effectiveness of interventions for ageing workers on (early) retirement, work ability and productivity: A systematic review. *International Archives of Occupational and Environmental Health*, August [Epub ahead of publication]. doi:10.1007/s00420-014-0969-y.

Coulson, M. 2013. *The Complete Guide to Personal Training*. London: Bloomsbury Sport.

Dunn, R. 1990. Understanding the Dunn and Dunn Learning Style Model and the need for individual diagnosis and prescription. *Journal of Reading, Writing, and Learning Disabilities* 6(3): 223–247.

Felder, R.M., and L.K. Silverman. 1988. Learning and teaching styles in engineering education. *Engineering Education* 78(7): 674–681.

Fleming, N. 2001. *Teaching and Learning Styles: VARK Strategies*. Christchurch, New Zealand: N.D. Fleming.

Fleming, N.D., and C. Mills. 1992. Not another inventory, rather a catalyst for reflection. *Improve the Academy* 11: 137.

Gregorc, A.F. 1979. Learning/teaching styles: Their nature and effects. In *Student learning styles*, edited by J.W. Keefe, 19-26. Reston, VA: National Association of Secondary School Principals.

Hawk, T.F., and A.J. Shah. 2007. Using learning style instruments to enhance student learning. *Decision Sciences Journal of Innovative Education* 5(1): 1–19.

Hutchison, A.J., J.D. Breckon, and L.H. Johnston. 2009. Physical activity behavior change interventions based on the transtheoretical model: A systematic review. *Health Education & Behavior* 36(5): 829–845. doi:10.1177/1090198108318491.

Irving, B.A., J. Rutkowski, D.W. Brock, C.K. Davis, E.J. Barrett, G.A. Gaesser et al. 2006. Comparison of Borg- and OMNI-RPE as markers of the blood lactate response to exercise. *Medicine & Science in Sports & Exercise* 38(7): 1348–1352. doi:10.1249/01.mss.0000227322.61964.d2.

Karageorghis, C.I., and D.L. Priest. 2012. Music in the exercise domain: A review and synthesis (part I). *International Review of Sport and Exercise Psychology* 5(1): 44–66. doi:10.1080/1750984X.2011.631026.

Kolb, D.A. 1984. *Experiential Learning: Experience as the Source of Learning and Development*. Englewood Cliffs, NJ: Prentice Hall.

Martin, S.B. 2013. Principles of behaviour change: Skill building to promote physical activity. In *ACSM's Resource Manual for Guidelines for Exercise Testing and Prescription*, edited by A.K. Swain, 745–760. Baltimore: Lippincott Williams & Wilkins.

McClanahan, B.S. 2013. Counselling physical activity behavior change. In *ACSM's Resource Manual for Guidelines for Exercise Testing and Prescription*, edited by A.K. Swain, 761–773. Baltimore: Lippincott Williams & Wilkins.

Napolitano, M.A. 2013. Theoretical foundations of physical activity behavior change. In *ACSM's Resource Manual for Guidelines for Exercise Testing and Prescription*, edited by A.K. Swain, 730–744. Baltimore: Lippincott Williams & Wilkins.

Persinger, R., C. Foster, M. Gibson, D.C. Fater, and J.P. Porcari. 2004. Consistency of the talk test for exercise prescription. *Medicine & Science in Sports & Exercise* 36(3): 533–553.

Prochaska, J.O., C.C. DiClemente, and J.C. Norcross. 1992. In search of how people change. Applications to addictive behaviors. *American Psychologist* 47(9): 1102–1114.

Ratey, J.J., and J.E. Loehr. 2011. The positive impact of physical activity on cognition during adulthood: A review of underlying mechanisms, evidence and recommendations. *Reviews in the Neurosciences* 22(2): 171–185. doi:10.1515/RNS.2011.017.

Riebe, D. 2013a. General principles of exercise prescription. In *ACSM's Guidelines for Exercise Testing and Prescription*, edited by L.S. Pescatello, 9th ed., 162–193. Baltimore: Lippincott Williams & Wilkins.

Riebe, D. 2013b. Behaviour theories and strategies for promoting exercise. In *ACSM's Guidelines for Exercise Testing and Prescription*, edited by L.S. Pescatello, 9th ed., 355–382. Baltimore: Lippincott Williams & Wilkins.

Schultz, A.B., and D.W. Edington. 2007. Employee health and presenteeism: A systematic review. *Journal of Occupational Rehabilitation* 17(3): 547–579. doi:10.1007/s10926-007-9096-x.

Silva, M.N., D. Markland, C.S. Minderico, P.N. Vieira, M.M. Castro, S.R. Coutinho et al. 2008. A randomized controlled trial to evaluate self-determination theory for exercise adherence and weight control: Rationale and intervention description. *BMC Public Health* 8: 234. doi:10.1186/1471-2458-8-234.

Spencer, L., T.B. Adams, S. Malone, L. Roy, and E. Yost. 2006. Applying the transtheoretical model to exercise: A systematic and comprehensive review of the literature. *Health Promotion Practice* 7(4): 428–443. doi:10.1177/1524839905278900.

Teixeira, P.J., E.V. Carraça, D. Markland, M.N. Silva, and R.M. Ryan. 2012. Exercise, physical activity, and self-determination theory: A systematic review. *International Journal of Behavioral Nutrition and Physical Activity* 9(1): 78.

Thompson, P.D. 2013. Participation health screening. In *ACSM's Guidelines for Exercise Testing and Prescription*, edited by L.S. Pescatello, 9th ed., 19–38. Baltimore: Lippincott Williams & Wilkins.

von Leupoldt, A., R. Ambruzsova, S. Nordmeyer, N. Jeske, and B. Dahme. 2006. Sensory and affective aspects of dyspnea contribute differentially to the Borg scale's measurement of dyspnea. *Respiration* 73(6): 762–768. doi:10.1159/000095910.

Chapter 4

Aaberg, E. 2006. *Muscle Mechanics*. 2nd ed. Champaign, IL: Human Kinetics.

Bear, M.F., B.W. Connor, and M.A. Paradiso. 2007. *Neuroscience: Exploring the Brain*. 3rd ed. Baltimore: Lippincott Williams & Wilkins.

Chandler, T.J., and L.E. Brown. 2006. *Conditioning for Strength and Human Performance*. Baltimore: Lippincott Williams & Wilkins.

Farrell, P.A., M.J. Joyner, J. Vincent, and V.J. Caiozzo. 2011. *ACSM's Advanced Exercise Physiology*. 2nd ed. Baltimore: Lippincott Williams & Wilkins.

Hall, S.J. 2014. *Basic Biomechanics*. New York: McGraw-Hill.

Hamill, J., K.M. Knutzen, and T.R. Derrick. 2014. *Biomechanical Basis of Human Movement*. Baltimore: Lippincott Williams & Wilkins.

Levangie, P.K, and C.C. Norkin. 2011. *Joint Structure and Function: A Comprehensive Analysis*. 5th ed. Philadelphia: F.A. Davis.

Moore, K.L., and A.F. Dalley. 2006. *Clinically Oriented Anatomy*. 5th ed. Baltimore: Lippincott Williams & Wilkins.

Nazarian, A.B, K. Khayambashi, and N. Rahnama. 2010. Dominant and non-dominant leg bone mineral density in professional soccer players and non-athlete subjects. *World Journal of Sport Sciences* 3(1): 28–32.

Nordin, M., and V. Frankel. 2012. *Basic Biomechanics of the Musculoskeletal System*. 4th ed. Baltimore: Lippincott Williams & Wilkins.

Salter, R.B. 1998. *Textbook of Disorders and Injuries of the Musculoskeletal System*. 3rd ed. Baltimore: Lippincott Williams & Wilkins.

Wakefield, R.J., and M.A. D'Agostino. 2010. *Essential Applications of Musculoskeletal Ultrasound in Rheumatology: Expert Consult Premium Edition*. Philadelphia: Saunders.

Ward, K. 2004. *Hands on Sports Therapy*. Boston: Cengage Learning.

Watkins, J. 2010. *Structure and Function of the Musculoskeletal System*. Champaign, IL: Human Kinetics.

Whiting, W., and S. Rugg. 2012. *Dynatomy: Dynamic Human Anatomy*. Champaign, IL: Human Kinetics.

Whiting, W.C., and R.F. Zernicke. 2008. *Biomechanics of Musculoskeletal Injury*. 2nd ed. Champaign, IL: Human Kinetics.

Chapter 5

Body, J.J., P. Bergmann, S. Boonen, Y. Boutsen, O. Bruyere, J.P. Devogalaer et al. 2011. Non-pharmacological management of osteoporosis: A consensus of the Belgian Bone Club. *Osteoporosis International* 22(11): 2769–2788.

Buckwalter, J.A. 1995. Aging and degeneration of the human intervertebral disc. *Spine* 20(11): 1307–1314.

Fong, D.T., Y.Y. Chan, K.M. Mok, P.Sh. Yung, and K.M. Chan. 2009. Understanding acute ankle ligamentous sprain injury in sports. *Sports Medicine, Arthroscopy, Rehabilitation, Therapy & Technology* 1: 14.

Friedlander A.L., H.K. Genant, S. Sadowsky, N.N. Byl, and C.C. Glüer. 1995. A two-year program of aerobics and weight training enhances bone mineral density of young women. *Journal of Bone and Mineral Research* 10(4): 574–585.

Fusco, C., F. Zaina, S. Atanasio, M. Romano, A. Negrini, and S. Negrini. 2011. Physical exercises in the treatment of adolescent idiopathic scoliosis: An updated systematic review. *Physiotherapy Theory and Practice* 27(1): 80–114.

Goss, T.P. 1988. Anterior glenohumeral instability. *Orthopedics* 11(1): 87–95.

Guo, Z., and R. De Vita. 2009. Probabilistic constitutive law for damage in ligaments. *Medical Engineering & Physics* 31(9): 1104–1109.

Harkness, E.F., G.J. Macfarlane, A.J. Silman, and J. McBeth. 2005. Is musculoskeletal pain more common now than 40 years ago? Two population-based cross-sectional studies. *Rheumatology (Oxford)* 44(7): 890–895.

Hodges, P.W., and C.A. Richardson. 1997. Contraction of the abdominal muscles associated with movement of the lower limb. *Physical Therapy* 77(2): 132–134.

Hodges, P.W., and C.A. Richardson. 1998. Delayed postural contraction of transversus abdominis in low back pain associated with movement of the lower limb. *Journal of Spinal Disorders* 11(1): 46–56.

Hootman, J.M., C.A. Macera, B.E. Ainsworth, C.L. Addy, M. Martin, and S.N. Blair. 2002. Epidemiology of musculoskeletal injuries among sedentary and physically active adults. *Medicine & Science in Sports & Exercise* 34(5): 838–844.

de Kam, D., E. Smulders, V. Weerdesteyn, and B.C. Smits-Engelsman. 2009. Exercise interventions to reduce fall-related fractures and their risk factors in individuals with low bone density: A systematic review of randomized controlled trials. *Osteoporosis International* 20(12): 2111–2125.

Kibler, W.B. 1989. The role of the scapula in athletic shoulder function. *American Journal of Sports Medicine* 26(2): 325–337.

Księżopolska-Orłowska, K. 2010. Changes in bone mechanical strength in response to physical therapy. *Polskie Archiwum Medycyny Wewnętrznej* 120(9): 368–373.

Layne, J.E., and M.E. Nelson. 1999. The effects of progressive resistance training on bone density: A review. *Medicine & Science in Sports & Exercise* 31(1): 25–30.

Lewis, C.B., and J.M. Bottomly. 2007. *Geriatric Rehabilitation. A Clinical Approach.* 3rd ed. Upper Saddle River, NJ: Prentice Hall.

Magkos, F., M. Yannakoulia, S.A. Kavouras, and L.S. Sidossis. 2007. The type and intensity of exercise have independent and additive effects on bone mineral density. *International Journal of Sports Medicine* 28(9): 773–779.

Nachemson, A.L. 1981. Disc pressure measurements. *Spine* 6(1): 93–97.

National Institutes of Health. 2000. Osteoporosis prevention, diagnosis and therapy. *NIH Consensus Statement 2000 March 27-29* 17(1): 1–45.

O'Sullivan, P.B., L. Twomey, and G. Allison. 1997. Evaluation of specific stabilizing exercises in the treatment of chronic low back pain with radiologic diagnosis of spondylosis or spondylolisthesis. *Spine* 22(24): 2959–2967.

Page, P., C. Frank, and R. Lardner. 2010. *Assessment and Treatment of Muscle Imbalance. The Janda Approach.* Champaign, IL: Human Kinetics.

Prokopy, M.P., C.D. Ingersoll, E. Nordenschild, F.I. Katch, G.A. Gaesser, and A. Weltman. 2008. Closed-kinetic chain upper-body training improves throwing performance of NCAA division I softball players. *Journal of Strength and Conditioning Research* 22(6): 1790–1798.

Sahrmann, S. 1993. Movement as a cause of musculoskeletal pain. *MPPA Conference Proceedings.* Perth, Australia.

Snow-Harter, C., M.L. Bouxsein, B.T. Lewis, D.R. Carter, and R. Marcus. 1992. Effects of resistance and endurance exercise on bone mineral status of young women. *Journal of Bone and Mineral Research* 7(7): 761–769.

Solomonow, M. 2009. Ligaments: A source of musculoskeletal disorders. *Journal of Body Work and Movement Therapies* 13(2): 136–154.

Verhagen, E., A. van der Beek, J. Twisk, L. Bouter, R. Bahr, and W. van Mechelen. 2004. The effect of a proprioceptive balance board training program for the prevention of ankle sprains. A prospective controlled trial. *American Journal of Sports Medicine* 32(6): 1385–1393.

Voight, M.L., and B.C. Thomson. 2000. The role of the scapula in the rehabilitation of shoulder injuries. *Journal of Athletic Training* 35(3): 364–372.

Chapter 6

Aagaard, P., J.L. Andersen, P. Dyhre-Poulsen, A.M. Leffers, A. Wagner, S.P. Magnusson et al. 2001. A mechanism for increased contractile strength of human pennate muscle in response to strength training: Changes in muscle architecture. *The Journal of Physiology* 534(Pt. 2): 613–623.

Bolster, D.R., L.S. Jefferson, and S.R. Kimball. 2004. Regulation of protein synthesis associated with skeletal muscle hypertrophy by insulin-, amino acid- and exercise-induced signalling. *The Proceedings of the Nutrition Society* 63(2): 351–356.

Bottinelli, R., S. Schiaffino, and C. Reggiani. 1991. Force-velocity relations and myosin heavy chain isoform compositions of skinned fibres from rat skeletal muscle. *The Journal of Physiology* 437(1): 655–672.

Bottinelli, R., M. Canepari, M.A. Pellegrino, and C. Reggiani. 1996. Force-velocity properties of human skeletal muscle fibres: Myosin heavy chain isoform and temperature dependence. *The Journal of Physiology* 495(2): 573–586.

Clark, M.G., S. Rattigan, E.J. Barrett, and M.A. Vincent. 2008. Point: Counterpoint: There is/is not capillary recruitment in active skeletal muscle during exercise. *Journal of Applied Physiology* 104(3): 889–891.

Enoka, R.M. 1996. Eccentric contractions require unique activation strategies by the nervous system. *Journal of Applied Physiology* 81(6): 2339–2346.

Gibala, M.J., and S.L. McGee. 2008. Metabolic adaptations to short-term high-intensity interval training. *Exercise and Sport Sciences Reviews* 36(2): 58–63.

Gordon, A.M., A.F. Huxley, and F.J. Julian. 1966. The variation in isometric tension with sarcomere length in vertebrate muscle fibres. *The Journal of Physiology* 184(1): 170–192.

Henneman, E., G. Somjen, and D.O. Carpenter. 1965. Excitability and inhibitability of motoneurons of different sizes. *Journal of Neurophysiology* 28(3): 599–620.

Holloszy, J.O., and E.F. Coyle. 1984. Adaptations of skeletal muscle to endurance exercise and their metabolic consequences. *Journal of Applied Physiology* 56(4): 831–838.

Joyner, M.J. 2006. Exercise hyperemia: Waiting for the reductionists? *American Journal of Physiology Heart and Circulatory Physiology* 291(3): H1032–H1033.

Knuttgen, H.G., and W.J. Kraemer. 1987. Terminology and measurement in exercise performance. *Journal of Strength and Conditioning Research* 1(1): 1.

Kraemer, W.J., K. Adams, E. Cafarelli, G.A. Dudley, C. Dooly, M.S. Feigenbaum et al. 2002. American College of Sports Medicine position stand. Progression models in resistance training for healthy adults. *Medicine and Science in Sports and Exercise* 34(2): 364–380.

LaStayo, P.C., D.J. Pierotti, J. Pifer, H. Hoppeler, and S.L. Lindstedt. 2000. Eccentric ergometry: Increases in locomotor muscle size and strength at low training intensities. *American Journal of Physiology—Regulatory, Integrative and Comparative Physiology* 278(5): R1282–R1288.

Lindstedt, S.L., P.C. LaStayo, and T.E. Reich. 2001. When active muscles lengthen: Properties and consequences of eccentric contractions. *Physiology* 16(6): 256–261.

McPhedran, A.M., R.B. Wuerker, and E. Henneman. 1965a. Properties of motor units in a heterogenous pale muscle (m. gastrocnemius) of the cat. *Journal of Neurophysiology* 28: 85–99.

McPhedran, A.M., R.B. Wuerker, and E. Henneman. 1965b. Properties of motor units in a heterogenous pale muscle (m. soleus) of the cat. *Journal of Neurophysiology* 28: 71–84.

Miller, B.F., J.L. Olesen, M. Hansen, S. Døssing, R.M. Crameri, R.J. Welling et al. 2005. Coordinated collagen and muscle protein synthesis in human patella tendon and quadriceps muscle after exercise. *The Journal of Physiology* 567(Pt 3): 1021–1033.

Phillips, S.M., K.D. Tipton, A.A. Ferrando, and R.R. Wolfe. 1999. Resistance training reduces the acute exercise-induced increase in muscle protein turnover. *The American Journal of Physiology* 276(1 Pt 1): E118–E124.

Poole, D.C., M.D. Brown, and O. Hudlicka. 2008. Counterpoint: There is not capillary recruitment in active skeletal muscle during exercise. *Journal of Applied Physiology* 104(3): 891–893.

Ryschon, T.W., M.D. Fowler, R.E. Wysong, A.R. Anthony, and R.S. Balaban. 1997. Efficiency of human skeletal muscle in vivo: Comparison of isometric, concentric, and eccentric muscle action. *Journal of Applied Physiology* 83(3): 867–874.

Schoenfeld, B.J. 2010. The mechanisms of muscle hypertrophy and their application to resistance training. *Journal of Strength and Conditioning Research* 24(10): 2857–2872.

Sheriff, D. 2005. Point: The muscle pump raises muscle blood flow during locomotion. *Journal of Applied Physiology* 99(1): 371–372.

Thorstensson, A., G. Grimby, and J. Karlsson. 1976. Force-velocity relations and fiber composition in human knee extensor muscles. *Journal of Applied Physiology* 40(1): 12–16.

Chapter 7

Achten, J., M. Gleeson, and A.E. Jeukendrup. 2002. Determination of the exercise intensity that elicits maximal fat oxidation. *Medicine & Science in Sports & Exercise* 34(1): 92–97.

Ainsworth, B.E., W.L. Haskell, S.D. Herrmann, N. Meckes, D.R. Bassett Jr., C. Tudor-Locke et al. 2011. Compendium of Physical Activities: A second update of codes and MET values. *Medicine & Science in Sports & Exercise* 43(8): 1575–1581.

American College of Sports Medicine (ACSM). 1998. The recommended quantity and quality of exercise for developing and maintaining cardiorespiratory and muscular fitness, and flexibility in healthy adults. *Medicine & Science in Sports & Exercise* 30(6): 975–991.

Borg, G. 1970. Perceived exertion as an indicator of somatic stress. *Scandinavian Journal of Rehabilitation Medicine* 2(2): 92–98.

Clark M.A., Lucett, S.C., and B.G. Sutton. 2011. *NASM Essentials of Personal Fitness Training* 4th ed. Baltimore: Lippincott, Williams and Wilkins.

Fox 3rd, S.M., Naughton, J.P., and W.L. Haskell. 1971. Physical activity and the prevention of coronary heart disease. *Annals of Clinical Research* 3(6): 404-432.

Jeukendrup, A., and J. Achten. 2001. Fatmax: A new concept to optimize fat oxidation during exercise. *European Journal of Sport Science* 1(5): 1–5.

Katch, V.L., McArdle, W.D., and F.I. Katch. 2010. *Essentials of Exercise Physiology.* 4th ed. Baltimore: Lippincott Williams & Wilkins.

Kenney, W.L., J. Wilmore, and D. Costill. 2011. *Physiology of Sport and Exercise.* 5th ed. Champaign, IL: Human Kinetics.

McArdle, W.D., Katch, F.I., and V. L. Katch 2005. *Essentials of Exercise Physiology.* Baltimore: Lippincott Williams & Wilkins.

Chapter 8

Anderson, R., D.E. Spicer, A. Hlavacek, A. Cook, and C. Backer. 2013. *Wilcox's Surgical Anatomy of the Heart.* Cambridge, England: Cambridge University Press.

Blair, S.N. 2009. Physical inactivity: The biggest public health problem of the 21st century. *British Journal of Sports Medicine* 43: 1–2.

Hogg, J.C., F. Chu, S. Utokaparch, R. Woods, W.M. Elliott, L. Buzatu, et al. 2004. The nature of small-airway obstruction in chronic obstructive pulmonary disease. *New England Journal of Medicine* 350: 2645–2653.

Klabunde, R.E. 2011. *Cardiovascular Physiology Concepts.* Baltimore: Lippincott Williams & Wilkins.

Pedersen, B.K., and B. Saltin. 2006. Evidence for prescribing exercise as therapy in chronic disease. *Scandinavian Journal of Medicine and Science in Sports* 16(Suppl 1): 3–63.

Rees, P.J., P.J. Chowienczyk, and T.J. Clark. 1982. Immediate response to cigarette smoke. *Thorax* 37(6): 417–422.

Smith, D., and B. Fernhall. 2010. *Advanced Cardiovascular Exercise Physiology.* Champaign, IL: Human Kinetics.

Standring, S. 2008. *Gray's Anatomy: The Anatomical Basis of Clinical Practice, Expert Consult.* 40th ed. London: Churchill Livingstone.

Chapter 9

Baechle, T.R., and E.W. Earle. 2008. *Essentials of Strength and Conditioning.* 3rd ed. Champaign, IL: Human Kinetics.

Bompa, T.O., and M.C. Carrera. 2005. *Periodization Training for Sports.* 2nd ed. Champaign, IL: Human Kinetics.

Brooks, G.A, T.D. Fahey, T.P. White, and K. Baldwin. 2008. *Exercise Physiology: Human Bioenergetics and Its Application.* 4th ed. New York: McGraw-Hill.

Clark, M.A., S.C. Lucett, and B.G. Sutton. 2012. *NASM Essentials of Personal Fitness Training.* 4th ed. Baltimore: Lippincott Williams & Wilkins.

Drury, D.G. 2000. Strength and proprioception. *Orthopedic Physical Therapy Clinic* 9(4): 549–561.

Fox, S.I. 2006. *Human Physiology.* 9th ed. New York: McGraw-Hill.

Gardiner, P.F. 2001. *Neuromuscular Aspects of Physical Activity.* Champaign, IL: Human Kinetics.

Grigg, P. 1994. Peripheral neural mechanisms in proprioception. *Journal of Sport Rehabilitation* 3: 2–17.

Hanes, D.A., and G. McCollum. 2006. Cognitive-vestibular interactions: A review of patient difficulties and possible mechanisms. *Journal of Vestibular Research* 16(3): 75–91.

Hoffman, J. 2002. *Physiological Aspects of Sport Training and Performance.* Champaign, IL: Human Kinetics.

Lephart, S.M., D. Pincivero, J. Giraldo, and F. Fu. 1997. The role of proprioception in the management and rehabilitation of athletic injuries. *American Journal of Sports Medicine* 25: 130–137.

Lodish H., A. Berk, S.L. Zipursky et al. 2000. *Molecular Cell Biology.* 4th ed. New York: W.H. Freeman.

McArdle, W., F. Katch, and V. Katch. 2005. *Essentials of Exercise Physiology.* Baltimore: Lippincott Williams & Wilkins.

Noback, C., D. Ruggiero, R. Demarest, and N. Strominger. 2005. *The Human Nervous System: Structure and Function.* 6th ed. New York: Humana Press.

Ratamess, N. 2012. *ACSM's Foundations of Strength Training and Conditioning.* Baltimore: Lippincott Williams & Wilkins.

Robbins, D., and E. Zeinstra. 2015. Muscle action. In *Europe Active's Foundations for Exercise Professionals,* edited by T. Rieger, F. Naclerio, A. Jiménez and J. Moody. Champaign, IL: Human Kinetics.

Tortora, G.J. 2001. *Principles of Human Anatomy.* 9th ed. New York: John Wiley & Sons.

Vander, A., J. Sherman, and D. Luciano. 2001. *Human Physiology: The Mechanisms of Body Function.* 8th ed. New York: McGraw-Hill.

Chapter 10

McArdle, W.D., F.I. Katch, and V.L. Katch. 2009. *Exercise Physiology.* 7th ed. Baltimore: Lippincott Williams & Wilkins.

Kraemer, W.J. 1988. Endocrine responses to resistance exercise. *Medicine & Science in Sports & Exercise* 2(5): S152-S157.

Chapter 11

American College of Sports Medicine (ACSM). 2007. *ACSM's Health-related Physical Fitness Assessment Manual.* 2nd ed. Baltimore: Lippincott Williams & Wilkins.

American College of Sports Medicine (ACSM). 2013. *ACSM's Health-related Physical Fitness Assessment Manual.* 4th ed. Baltimore: Lippincott Williams & Wilkins.

Arena, R. (2013). Health-Related Physical Fitness Testing and Interpretation. In L. S. Pescatello (Ed.), *ACSM's Guidelines for Exercise Testing and Prescription* (9th ed., pp. 60–113). Baltimore: Lippincott, Williams & Wilkins.

Baechle, T.R., and R.W. Earle. 2008. *Essentials of Strength Training and Conditioning.* 3rd ed. Champaign, IL: Human Kinetics.

Beekley, M. D., Brechue, W. F., Dehoyos, D. V., Garzarella, L., Werber-Zion, G., & Pollock, M. L. (2004). Cross-validation of the YMCA submaximal cycle ergometer test to predict $\dot{V}O_2$max. *Research Quarterly for Exercise and Sport,* 75(3), 337–342. http://doi.org/10.1080/02701367.2004.10609165.

Bruce, R. A. (1971). Exercise testing of patients with coronary heart disease. Principles and normal standards for evaluation. *Ann Clin Res*, 3(6), 323–32.

Brzycki, M. 1998. *A Practical Approach to Strength Training*. 3rd ed. New York: McGraw-Hill.

Canadian Society for Exercise Physiology. (2013). Canadian Society for Exercise Physiology-Physical Activity Training for Health (CSEP-PATH). Ottawa, ON.: Canadian Society for Exercise Physiology.

Caspersen, C.J., K.E. Powell, and G.M. Christenson. 1985. Physical activity, exercise, and physical fitness: Definitions and distinctions for health-related research. *Public Health Reports* 100(2): 126–131.

Centers for Disease Control (CDC). 1996. *Physical Activity and Health: A Report of the Surgeon General*. Atlanta: Author.

Chobanian, A.V., G.L. Bakris, H.R. Black, W.C. Cushman, L.A. Green, J.L. Izzo Jr. et al. 2003. The Seventh Report of the Joint National Committee on Prevention, Detection, Evaluation, and Treatment of High Blood Pressure: The JNC 7 report. *JAMA* 289(19): 2560–2572.

Costa, J., M. Borges, E. Oliveira, M. Gouveia, and A.V. Carneiro. 2003. Incidence and prevalence of hypercholesterolemia in Portugal: A systematic review. Part I. *Revista Portuguesa de Cardiologia* 22(4): 569–577.

Fields, L., Burt, V., Cutler, J., Hughes, J., Roccella, E., & Sorlie, P. (2004). The Burden of Adult Hypertension in the United States 1999 to 2000. A Rising Tide. *Hypertension*, 44, 398–404.

Greenland, P., Alpert, J. S., Beller, G. A., Benjamin, E. J., Budoff, M. J., Fayad, Z. A., ... Jacobs, A. K. (2010). 2010 ACCF/AHA Guideline for Assessment of Cardiovascular Risk in Asymptomatic Adults: Executive Summary: A Report of the American College of Cardiology Foundation/American Heart Association Task Force on Practice Guidelines. *Circulation*, 122(25), 2748–2764. http://doi.org/10.1161/CIR.0b013e3182051bab.

Haqq, A.M., D.S. DeLorey, A.M. Sharma, M. Freemark, F. Kreier, M.L. Mackenzie et al. 2012. Autonomic nervous system dysfunction in obesity and Prader-Willi syndrome: Current evidence and implications for future obesity therapies. *Clinical Obesity* 1(4-6): 175–183.

Heyward, V.H. 2010. *Advanced Fitness Assessment and Exercise Prescription*. 6th ed. Champaign, IL: Human Kinetics.

Iglesias-Soler, E., and M. Chapman. 2015. Components and principles of fitness. In *EuropeActive's Foundations for Exercise Professionals*, edited by T. Rieger, F. Naclerio, A. Jiménez, and J. Moody. Champaign, IL: Human Kinetics.

Jurca, R., Jackson, A. S., LaMonte, M. J., Morrow, J. R., Blair, S. N., Wareham, N. J., ... Laukkanen, R. (2005). Assessing Cardiorespiratory Fitness Without Performing Exercise Testing. *American Journal of Preventive Medicine*, 29(3), 185–193. http://doi.org/10.1016/j.amepre.2005.06.004

Kamel, E.G., G. McNeill, and M.C. Van Wijk. 2000. Usefulness of anthropometry and DXA in predicting intra-abdominal fat in obese men and women. *Obesity Research* 8(1): 36–42.

Kline, G.M., J.P. Porcari, R. Hintermeister, P.S. Freedson, A. Ward, R.F. McCarron et al. 1987. Estimation of $\dot{V}O_2$max from a one-mile track walk, gender, age, and body weight. *Medicine and Science in Sports and Exercise* 19(3): 253–259.

Lohman, T.G., and Z. Chen. 2005. Dual-energy X-ray absorptiometry. In *Human Body Composition*, edited by S.B. Heymsfield, T.G. Lohman, Z. Wang, and S. Going. Champaign, IL: Human Kinetics.

Lombardi, V. 1989. *Beginning Weight Training*. Dubuque, IA: Brown.

MacDougall, J.D., H.A. Wenger, and H.J. Green, eds. 1991. *Physiological Testing of the High-Performance Athlete*. Champaign, IL: Human Kinetics.

McArdle, W.D., F.I. Katch, G.S. Pechar, L. Jacobson, and S. Ruck. 1972. Reliability and interrelationships between maximal oxygen intake, physical work capacity and step-test scores in college women. *Medicine and Science in Sports* 4(4): 182–186.

Moody, J., and R. Stevens. 2015. Screening and assessing. In *EuropeActive's Foundations for Exercise Professionals*, edited by T. Rieger, F. Naclerio, A. Jiménez, and J. Moody. Champaign, IL: Human Kinetics.

National Institutes of Health (NIH). 1997. The sixth report of the Joint National Committee on prevention, detection, evaluation, and treatment of high blood pressure. *Archives of Internal Medicine* 157(21): 2413–2446.

Page, P., Frank, C., & Lardner, R. (2010). *Assessment and Treatment of Muscle Imbalance* (1 edition). Champaign, IL: Human Kinetics.

Park, Y.W., S.B. Heymsfield, and D. Gallagher. 2002. Are dual-energy X-ray absorptiometry regional estimates associated with visceral adipose tissue mass? *International Journal of Obesity and Related Metabolism Disorders* 26(7): 978–983.

Perloff, D., C. Grim, J. Flack, E.D. Frohlich, M. Hill, M. McDonald et al. 1993. Human blood pressure determination by sphygmomanometry. *Circulation* 88(5): 2460–2470.

Riganello, F., G. Dolce, and W. Sannita. 2012. Heart rate variability and the central autonomic network in the severe disorder of consciousness. *Journal of Rehabilitation Medicine* 44(6): 495–501.

Santos-Rocha, R., and N. Pimenta. 2015. Safe and effective exercise. In *EuropeActive's Foundations for Exercise Professionals*, edited by T. Rieger, F. Naclerio, A. Jiménez, and J. Moody. Champaign, IL: Human Kinetics.

Sardinha, L.B., and P.J. Teixeira. 2005. Measuring adiposity and fat distribution in relation to health. In *Human Body Composition*, 2nd ed., edited by S.B. Heymsfield, T.G. Lohman, Z. Wang, and S.B. Going. Champaign, IL: Human Kinetics.

Seals, D.R. 2006. The autonomic nervous system. In *ACSM's Advanced Exercise Physiology*, edited by C.M. Tipton. Baltimore: Lippincott Williams & Wilkins.

Shen, W., Wang, Z., Punyanita, M., Lei, J., Sinav, A., Kral, J. G., ... Heymsfield, S. B. (2003). Adipose tissue quantification by imaging methods: a proposed classification. *Obes Res*, 11(1), 5–16.

Shen, W., M. St-Onge, Z. Wang, and S. Heymsfield. 2005. Study of body composition: An overview. In *Human Body Composition*, 2nd ed., edited by S. Heymsfield, T.G. Lohman, Z. Wang, and S. Going. Champaign, IL: Human Kinetics.

Thompson, P D. 2013. Benefits and risks associated with physical activity. In *ACSM's Guidelines for Exercise Testing and Prescription*, 9th ed., edited by L.S. Pescatello. Baltimore: Lippincott, Williams & Wilkins.

Vague, J. 1950. [Importance of the measurement of fat distribution in pathology.] *Bulletins et Memoires de la Societe Medicale des Hopitaux de Paris* 66(31-32): 1572–1574.

Vague, J. 1956. The degree of masculine differentiation of obesities: A factor determining predisposition to diabetes, atherosclerosis, gout, and uric calculous disease. *American Journal of Clinical Nutrition* 4(1): 20–34.

Wang, Z.M., R.N. Pierson Jr., and S.B. Heymsfield. 1992. The five-level model: A new approach to organizing body-composition research. *American Journal of Clinical Nutrition* 56(1): 19–28.

Weiglein, L., J. Herrick, S. Kirk, and E.P. Kirk. 2011. The 1-mile walk test is a valid predictor of $\dot{V}O_2$max and is a reliable alternative fitness test to the 1.5-mile run in US Air Force males. *Military Medicine* 176(6): 669–673.

Widmaier, E.P., H. Raff, and K.T. Strang. 2011. Structure of the nervous system. In *Vander's Human Physiology. The Mechanisms of Body Function*, 12th ed., edited by E.P. Widmaier, H. Raff, and K.T. Strang. New York: McGraw-Hill.

Widrick, J., Ward, A., Ebbeling, C., Clemente, E., & Rippe, J. M. (1992). Treadmill validation of an over-ground walking test to predict peak oxygen consumption. *European Journal of Applied Physiology and Occupational Physiology*, 64(4), 304–308.

Wilmore, J.H., and D.L. Costill. 2004. *Physiology of Sport and Exercise*. 3rd ed. Champaign, IL: Human Kinetics.

World Health Organization. 2009. Basic documents ; including amendments adopted up to 31st May 2009. Geneva: World Health Organization.

World Health Organization (WHO). 2003. 2003 World Health Organization (WHO)/International Society of Hypertension (ISH) statement on management of hypertension. *Journal of Hypertension* 21(11): 1983–1992.

Chapter 12

Anshel, M.H. 2014. *Applied Health Fitness Psychology*. Champaign, IL: Human Kinetics.

Beedie, C.J., A.N. Lane, and M.G. Wilson. 2012. A possible role for emotion and emotion regulation in physiological responses to false performance feedback in 10 mile laboratory cycling. *Applied Psychophysiology Biofeedback* 37(4): 269–277.

Comer, R.J. 2012. *Abnormal Psychology*. 8th ed. New York: Worth.

McCarney, R., J. Warner, S. Iliffe, R. van Haselen, M. Griffin, and P. Fisher. 2007. The Hawthorne Effect: A randomised, controlled trial. *BMC Medical Research Methodology* 7: 30.

Siegert, R.J., and W.J. Taylor. 2004. Theoretical aspects of goal-setting and motivation in rehabilitation. *Disability & Rehabilitation* 26(1): 1–8.

Weinberg, R.S., and D. Gould. 2011. *Foundations of Sport and Exercise Psychology*. 5th ed. Champaign, IL: Human Kinetics.

Chapter 13

Atkins, R.C. 1998. *Dr. Atkins' New Diet Revolution*. New York: Avon Books.

Bellisle, F., R. McDevitt, and A.M. Prentice. 1997. Meal frequency and energy balance. *The British Journal of Nutrition* 77(1): S57–S70.

Bohé, J., A. Low, R.R. Wolfe, and M.J. Rennie. 2003. Human muscle protein synthesis is modulated by extracellular, not intramuscular amino acid availability: A dose-response study. *The Journal of Physiology* 552(Pt 1): 315–324.

Børsheim, E., K.D. Tipton, S.E. Wolf, and R.R. Wolfe. 2002. Essential amino acids and muscle protein recovery from resistance exercise. *American Journal of Physiology, Endocrinology and Metabolism* 283(4): E648–E657.

Brooks, G.A., T.D. Fahey, and K.M. Baldwin. 2004. *Nutrition and Athletic Performance*. In *Exercise Physiology*, edited by G.A. Brooks, T.D. Fahey, and K.M. Baldwin. New York: McGraw Hill.

Burke, L.M., A.B. Loucks, and N. Broad. 2006. Energy and carbohydrate for training and recovery. *Journal of Sports Sciences* 24(7): 675–685.

Campbell, B., R.B. Kreider, T. Ziegenfuss, P. La Bounty, M. Roberts, D. Burke et al. 2007. International Society of Sports Nutrition position stand: Protein and exercise. *Journal of the International Society of Sports Nutrition* 4: 8.

Cunningham, J.J. 1980. A reanalysis of the factors influencing basal metabolic rate in normal adults. *The American Journal of Clinical Nutrition* 33(11): 2372–2374.

Dangin, M., C. Guillet, C. Garcia-Rodenas, P. Gachon, C. Bouteloup-Demange, K. Reiffers-Magnani et al. 2003. The rate of protein digestion affects protein gain differently during aging in humans. *Journal of Physiology* 549(Pt 2): 635–644.

Dansinger, M.L., J.A. Gleason, J.L. Griffith, H.P. Selker, and E.J. Schaefer. 2005. Comparison of the Atkins, Ornish, Weight Watchers, and Zone diets for weight loss and heart disease risk reduction. A randomized trial. *JAMA* 293(1): 43–53.

Dietary Guidelines Advisory Committee. 2010. *Report of the DGAC on the Dietary Guidelines for Americans* (Part D. Section 7: Alcohol D7-1 D7-24). Washington, DC: DGAC.

Eriksen M., Mackay J., & Ross H. 2012, *The Tobacco Atlas.* 4th Edition. American Cancer Society and World Lung Foundation.

Fontani, G., F. Corradeschi, A. Felici, F. Alfatti, R. Bugarini, A.I. Fiaschi et al. 2005. Blood profiles, body fat and mood state in healthy subjects on different diets supplemented with Omega-3 polyunsaturated fatty acids. *European Journal of Clinical Investigation* 35(8): 499–507.

Foster-Powell, K., S.A. Holt, and C.B. Brand-Miller. 2002. International table of glycemic index and glycemic load values. *The American Journal of Clinical Nutrition* 76(1): 5–56.

Goldstein, E.R., T. Ziegenfuss, D. Kalman, R. Kreider, B. Campbell, C. Wilborn et al. 2010. International Society of Sports Nutrition position stand: Caffeine and performance. *Journal of the International Society of Sports Nutrition* 7(1): 5.

Gómez Candela, C., L.M. Bermejo López, and V. Loria Kohenratio. 2011. Importance of a balanced omega 6/omega 3 ratio for the maintenance of health. *Nutrición Hospitalaria* 26(2): 323–329.

Harris, J., and F.A. Benedict. 1918. A biometric study of human basal metabolism. *Proceedings of the National Academy of Sciences USA* 4(12): 370–373.

Helge, J.E., W. Bolette, and B. Kiens. 1998. Impact of fat-rich diet on endurance in man: Role of the dietary period. *Medicine & Science in Sports & Exercise* 30(3): 456–461.

Ivy, J., and R. Portman. 2004. *Nutrient Timing.* Laguna Beach, CA: Basic Health.

Iwao, S., K. Mori, and Y. Sato. 1996. Effects of meal frequency on body composition during weight control in boxers. *Scandinavian Journal of Medicine & Science in Sports* 6(5): 265–272.

Jeukendrup, A.E., and M. Gleeson. 2010. *Sport Nutrition: An Introduction to Energy Production and Performance.* 2nd ed. Champaign, IL: Human Kinetics.

Kleiner, S.M. 2008. Nutritional assessment and counseling of athletes. In *Essentials of Sports Nutrition and Supplements,* edited by J. Antonio et al. New York: Humana Press.

La Bounty, P.M., B.I. Campbell, J. Wilson, E. Galvan, J. Berardi, S.M. Kleiner et al. 2011. International Society of Sports Nutrition position stand: Meal frequency. *Journal of the International Society of Sports Nutrition* 8: 4.

Layman, D.K., R.A. Boileau, D.J. Erickson, J.E. Painter, H. Shiue, C. Sather et al. 2003. A reduced ratio of dietary carbohydrate to protein improves body composition and blood lipid profiles during weight loss in adult women. *Journal of Nutrition* 133(2): 411–417.

Layman, D.K., and J.I. Baum. 2004. Dietary protein impact on glycemic control during weight loss. *Journal of Nutrition* 134(4): 968S–973S.

Layman, D.K., E.M. Evans, D. Erickson, J. Seyler, J. Weber, D. Bagshaw et al. 2009. A moderate-protein diet produces sustained weight loss and long-term changes in body composition and blood lipids in obese adults. *Journal of Nutrition* 139(3): 514–521.

Leddy, J., P. Horvath, J. Rowland, and D. Pendergast. 1997. Effect of a high or a low fat diet on cardiovascular risk factors in male and female runners. *Medicine & Science in Sports & Exercise* 29(1): 17–25.

Manore, M., and J. Thompson. 2000. *Sport Nutrition for Health and Performance.* Champaign, IL: Human Kinetics.

McArdle, W., F.I. Katch, and V.L. Katch. 2011. *Essentials of Exercise Physiology.* 4th ed. Baltimore: Lippincott Williams & Wilkins.

Naclerio, A.F. 2005. Nutrición y control del peso corporal. In *Entrenamiento Personal, Bases Fundamentos y Aplicaciones,* edited by A. Jiménez. Barcelona: Inde.

Naclerio, F., and J. Figueroa Alchapar. 2011. Organizacion de la dieta para personas sanas y deportistas. In *Entrenamiento Deportivo, Fundamentos y Aplicaciones en Diferentes Deportes,* edited by F. Naclerio. Madrid: Medica Panamericana.

Poehlman, E.T., and C. Melby. 1998. Resistance training and energy balance. *International Journal of Sport Nutrition* 8(2): 143–159.

Reimers, K. 2008. Nutritional factors in health and performance. In *Essentials of Strength Training and Conditioning,* edited by T.R. Baechle and R.W. Earle. Champaign, IL: Human Kinetics.

Riley, R.E. 1999. Popular weight loss diets. Health and exercise implication. *Clinics in Sports Medicine* 18(3): 691–701.

Roberts, S.B. 2000. High-glycemic index foods, hunger, and obesity: Is there a connection? *Nutrition Reviews* 58(6): 163–169.

Rodriguez, N.R., N.M. Di Marco, and S. Langley. 2009. ACSM position stand. Nutrition and athletes performance. *Medicine & Science in Sports & Exercise* 41(3): 709–731.

Ruidavets, J.B., V. Bongard, V. Bataille, P. Gourdy, and J. Ferrières. 2002. Eating frequency and body fatness in middle-aged men. *International Journal of Obesity and Related Metabolism Disorders* 26(11): 1476–1483.

Sears, B., and B. Lawren. 1995. *Enter the Zone.* New York: Regan Books.

Shugarman, A.E. 2008. A different look at the food guide pyramid. In *Essentials of Sports Nutrition and Supplements,* edited by J. Antonio et al. New York: Humana Press.

Simopoulos, A.P. 1991. Omega 3 fatty acid in health and disease and in growth and development. *The American Journal of Clinical Nutrition* 54(3): 438–463.

Simopoulos, A.P. 2002. Omega-3 fatty acids in inflammation and autoimmune diseases. *Journal of the American College of Nutrition* 21(6): 495–505.

Simopoulos, A.P. 2008. The omega-6/omega-3 fatty acid ratio, genetic variation, and cardiovascular disease. *Asia Pacific Journal of Clinical Nutrition* 17(1): 131–134.

Simopoulos, A.P. 2010. Evolutionary aspects of diet: The Omega-6/Omega-3 ratio and the brain. *Molecular Neurobiology* 44(2): 203–215.

U.S. Department of Health and Human Services. 2010. How Tobacco Smoke Causes Disease: The Biology and Behavioral Basis for Smoking-Attributable Disease. *A Report of the Surgeon General.* Atlanta, GA: U.S. Department of Health and Human Services.

Volek, J.S., J.L. Vanheest, and C.E. Forsythe. 2005. Diet and exercise for weight loss: A review of current issues. *Sports Medicine* 35(1): 1-9.

Volpe, S.L. 2006. Popular weight reduction diets. *Journal of Cardiovascular Nursing* 21(1): 34–39.

Williams, M.H. 2005. *Nutrition for Health, Fitness and Sport.* 7th ed. New York: McGraw-Hill.

Wolever, T.M.S. 2006. *Indice Glucémico. Clasificación fisiológica de los hidratos de carbono de la dieta.* Zaragoza, Spain: Acriba.

Ziegenfuss, T.N., J. Landis, and R.A. Lemieux. 2010. Protein for sports: New data and new recommendations. *Strength & Conditioning Journal* 32(1): 65–70.

Chapter 14

American College of Sport Medicine (ACSM). 2007. ACSM's Resources for the Personal Trainer. 2nd ed. Baltimore: Lippincott Williams & Wilkins.

American College of Sports Medicine (ACSM). 2012. *ACSM's Foundations of Strength Training and Conditioning.* Baltimore: Lippincott Williams & Wilkins.

American College of Sports Medicine. 2013. *ACSM's Guidelines for Exercise Testing and Prescription.* 9th ed. Baltimore: Lippincott Williams & Wilkins.

Baechle, T.R. and R.W. Earle. 2008. *Essentials of Strength Training and Conditioning.* 3rd ed. Champaign, IL: Human Kinetics.

Brooks, G.A. 1986. The lactate shuttle during exercise and recovery. *Medicine and Science in Sports and Exercise* 18(3): 360–368.

Gellish, R.L., B.R. Goslin, R.E. Olson, A. McDonald, G.D. Russi, and V.K. Moudgil. 2007. Longitudinal modeling of the relationship between age and maximal heart rate. *Medicine and Science in Sports and Exercise* 39(5): 822–829.

Hurley, B. 1994. Does strength training improve health status? *Strength & Conditioning* 16(3): 7–13.

Hurley, B., J.M. Hagberg, A.P. Goldberg, D.R. Seals, A.A. Ehsani, R.E. Brennan, and J.O. Holloszy. 1988. Resistance training can reduce coronary risk factors without altering $\dot{V}O_2$max or percent body fat. *Medicine and Science in Sports and Exercise* 20(2): 150–154.

Magel, J.R., G.F. Foglia, W.D. McArdle, B. Gutin, G.S. Pechar, and F.I. Katch. 1975. Specificity of swim training on maximum oxygen uptake. *Journal of Applied Physiology* 38(1): 151–155.

Maughan, R.J. 2009. *Olympic Textbook of Science in Sport.* Chichester, England: Wiley-Blackwell.

Reilly, T., N. Secher, P. Snell, and C. Williams. 1990. *Physiology of Sports.* Abingdon, England: Taylor & Francis.

Westcott, W. 1986. Integration of strength, endurance, and skill training. *Scholastic Coach* (May-June) 55: 74.

Westcott, W. 1993. Strength training and blood pressure response. *Nautilus* 2(4): 8–9.

Westcott, W. 1995. *Strength Fitness: Physiological Principles and Training Techniques.* 4th ed. Dubuque, IA: Brown and Benchmark.

Chapter 15

American College of Sports Medicine (ACSM). 2011. *ACSM's Foundations of Strength and Conditioning.* Baltimore: Lippincott Williams & Wilkins.

Benvenuti, P., and S. Zanuso. 2015. Cardiorespiratory exercise. In *EuropeActive's Foundations for Exercise Professionals,* edited by T. Rieger, F. Naclerio, A. Jiménez, and J. Moody. Champaign, IL: Human Kinetics.

Brzycki, M. 1998. *A Practical Approach to Strength Training.* 4th ed. Indianapolis, IN: McGraw-Hill.

Delorme, T.L., and A.L. Watkins. 1948. Technics of progressive resistance exercise. *Archives of Physical Medicine and Rehabilitation* 29(5): 263–273.

Fleck, S.J., and W.J. Kraemer. 2014. *Designing Resistance Training Programs.* 4th ed. Champaign, IL: Human Kinetics.

Klein, V. 1997. *Der Privat-Trainer.* Arnsberg, Germany: Novegenics.

Kraemer, W.J., and S.J. Fleck. 2007. *Optimizing Strength Training: Designing Nonlinear Periodization Workouts.* Champaign, IL: Human Kinetics.

Pedersen, B.K. 2011. Muscles and their myokines. *The Journal of Experimental Biology* 214(Pt 2): 337–346.

Pedersen, L., and P. Hojman. 2012. Muscle-to-organ cross talk mediated by myokines. *Adipocyte* 1(3): 164–167.

Peterson, M.D., M.R. Rhea, and B.A. Alvar. 2004. Maximizing strength development in athletes: A meta-analysis to determine the dose-response relationship. *Journal of Strength and Conditioning Research* 18(3): 377–382.

Ratamess, N.A., B.A. Alvar, T.K. Evetoch, T.J. Housh, B. Kibler, W.J. Kraemer et al. 2009. American College of Sports Medicine position stand. Progression models in resistance training for healthy adults. *Medicine and Science in Sports and Exercise* 41(3): 687–708.

Rhea, M.R., B.A. Alvar, L.N. Burkett, and S.D. Ball. 2003. A meta-analysis to determine the dose response for strength development. *Medicine and Science in Sports and Exercise* 35(3): 456–464.

Selye, H. 1950. *The Physiology and Pathology of Exposure to Stress. A Treatise Based on the Concepts of the General Adaptation Syndrome and the Diseases of Adaptation.* Montreal: Acta.

Siff, M.C. 2003. *Supertraining.* 6th ed. Denver: Supertraining Institute.

Starrett, K., and G. Cordoza. 2013. *Becoming a Supple Leopard: The Ultimate Guide to Resolving Pain, Preventing Injury, and Optimizing Athletic Performance.* Las Vegas, NV: Victory Belt.

Zatsiorsky, V.M., and W.J. Kraemer. 2006. *Science and Practice of Strength Training.* 2nd ed. Champaign, IL: Human Kinetics.

Index

Page numbers ending in an *f* or *t* indicate a figure or table, respectively.

About the Editors

Thomas Rieger, Dr. Rer. Soc., has been the chairman of the standards council of EuropeActive from 2012 to 2015. He holds a doctoral degree in social sciences with a specialization in sport science (German PhD equivalent) from the University of Tübingen and a master's degree in public health. In 2007, he was appointed as a professor of sport management at the Business and Information Technology School (BiTS) in Iserlohn, Germany. At BiTS, he is the vice dean of the bachelor's programme of sport and event management and the master's programme of international sport and event management. Previously, Dr. Rieger served as visiting professor at the Real Madrid Graduate School and the European University Cyprus in Nicosia. Before entering academia in 2006, he gained more than six years of experience in the fitness industry, especially in the fields of fitness marketing and quality management.

Ben Jones, BSc (Hons), is a founder and director of BlueSkies Fitness Ltd., a company that provides workplace wellness solutions to small and medium-sized employers, offers learning and development consultancy, and manages the process of training provider accreditation for EuropeActive. Mr. Jones has extensive experience of developing standards, qualifications, assessments and learning resources in the UK, Europe, and UAE and has written for EuropeActive, Active IQ, VTCT, Lifetime Awarding, and others. He is a master trainer for MEND, Momenta, and TechnoGym, and was one of the first PTA global faculty in the UK. Previously, he held the role of teaching and curriculum manager at Lifetime Training. Prior to entering the fitness sector in 1999 and going on to build a successful personal training practice and hold multiple fitness management roles, Mr. Jones studied physiology at Leeds University.

Alfonso Jiménez, PhD, CSCS, NSCA-CPT, FLF, is a professor of exercise science and health and the executive director of the Centre for Applied Biological and Exercise Sciences at Coventry University (UK), and a member of the scientific advisory board of UKActive Research Institute. Previous roles include professor and dean of the faculty of health, exercise and sports science at European University of Madrid (Spain), and main academic leader of the Real Madrid

Graduate School; professor, deputy dean and head of school of sport and exercise science at Victoria University in Melbourne (Australia); professor and head of the centre for sport science & human performance at the University of Greenwich in London (UK); and chairman of the standards council at EuropeActive. He was awarded honorary membership of EuropeActive in recognition of his outstanding service. He is currently serving as visiting professor and international research associate at ISEAL, Victoria University, visiting professor at the University of Greenwich, and chair of the research and dissemination commission at the Healthy & Active Living Foundation in Spain. Dr. Jiménez's background before entering academia centred on the fitness industry in management, research and sales.

Contributors

Christoffer Andersen
Fit&Sund, Denmark

Lars L. Andersen
Aalborg University, Faculty of Medicine, Department of Health Science and Technology, Denmark

Alexis Batrakoulis
GRAFTS, Greek Aerobics and Fitness Training School, Greece

Chris Beedie
University of Essex, United Kingdom

Francesco Bertiato
Technogym, Italy

João Brito
ESDRM-IPS, *Escola Superior de Desporto de Rio Maior - Instituto Politécnico de Santarém* (Sport Sciences School of Rio Maior - Polytechnic Institute of Santarém), Portugal

Cedric X. Bryant
American Council on Exercise, United States

Robert Cooper
University of Greenwich, Department of Life and Sports Sciences, United Kingdom

Davide Filingeri
University of Sydney, Australia

Mark Goss-Sampson
University of Greenwich, Department of Life and Sports Sciences, United Kingdom

Pauline Jacobs
HAN University of Applied Sciences, Nijmegen, The Netherlands

Ben Jones
Blueskies Fitness, United Kingdom

Samantha Jones
Blueskies Fitness, United Kingdom

Sabrena Merrill
American Council on Exercise, United States

Jan Middelkamp
HDD Group, The Netherlands

Fernando Naclerio
University of Greenwich, Department of Life and Sports Sciences, United Kingdom

Anders Nedergaard
Nordic Bioscience, Denmark

Rafael Oliveira
ESDRM-IPS, *Escola Superior de Desporto de Rio Maior - Instituto Politécnico de Santarém* (Sport Sciences School of Rio Maior - Polytechnic Institute of Santarém), Portugal

Nuno Pimenta
ESDRM-IPS, *Escola Superior de Desporto de Rio Maior - Instituto Politécnico de Santarém* (Sport Sciences School of Rio Maior - Polytechnic Institute of Santarém), Portugal

Thomas Rieger
BiTS, Business and Information Technology School, Faculty of International Service Industries, Germany

Daniel Robbins
University of Bedfordshire, United Kingdom

Simonetta Senni
Technogym, Italy

John van Heel
EFAA, The Netherlands

About EuropeActive

The European Register of Exercise Professionals uses the EuropeActive standards as its quality assurance process to ensure that exercise professionals are suitably qualified to offer safe and effective fitness programmes to their clients all across Europe. EREPS provides consumers, employers and partners in medical professions with the necessary level of confidence that registered trainers are competent and work to support its Code of Ethical Practice which defines the rights and principles of being an exercise professional. By referencing the EuropeActive standards to each trainer and by being registered it means that they have met the prescribed minimum standards of good practice, that they are committed to raising their standards, skills and professional status through a process of lifelong learning.

EREPS is regulated by the EuropeActive Standards Council using the accepted official European Qualification Framework which describes the knowledge, skills and competencies exercise professionals need to achieve for registration.

About the EuropeActive Series

Endorsed by EuropeActive, the continent's leading standard-setting organisation in fitness and health, these texts are the authoritative guides for current and future exercise professionals and training providers in Europe.

Authored by renowned experts from all over Europe, the information in these texts ranges from foundational knowledge to specific practical essentials for exercise professionals. For those who promote physical activity and healthier lifestyles, there are no other titles with more authority in Europe.

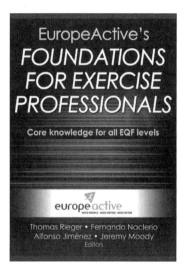

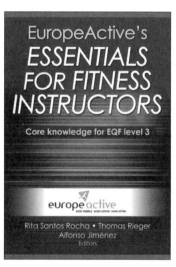

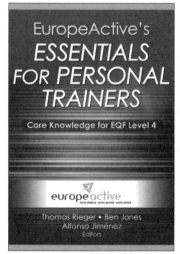

EuropeActive's Foundations for Exercise Professionals
EuropeActive
Thomas Rieger,
Fernando Naclerio,
Alfonso Jiménez, and
Jeremy Moody, Editors
©2015 • Hardback • 352 pp
Print: ISBN 978-1-4504-2377-9
E-book: ISBN 978-1-4925-0577-8

EuropeActive's Essentials for Fitness Instructors
EuropeActive
Rita Santos Rocha,
Thomas Rieger, and
Alfonso Jiménez, Editors
©2015 • Hardback • 208 pp
Print: ISBN 978-1-4504-2379-3
E-book: ISBN 978-1-4925-0591-4

EuropeActive's Essentials for Personal Trainers
EuropeActive
Thomas Rieger, Ben Jones,
and Alfonso Jiménez, Editors
©2016 • Hardback
Approx. 328 pp
Print: ISBN 978-1-4504-2378-6
E-book: ISBN 978-1-4925-2580-6

Find out more at www.HumanKinetics.com!

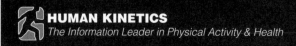

HUMAN KINETICS
The Information Leader in Physical Activity & Health

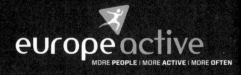

europe active
MORE PEOPLE | MORE ACTIVE | MORE OFTEN